Silencing the
Cough

Dry Cough symptoms
And Natural Home
Remedies

Dr. Harry Rusden

Copyright © 2024 Dr. Harry Rusden
Alright reserved

Table of Contents

I. Introduction to Dry Cough
   A. Definition and Characteristics
   B. Causes of Dry Cough
   C. Common Symptoms Associated with Dry Cough

II. Understanding the Importance of Treating Dry Cough
   A. Impact on Quality of Life
   B. Potential Complications of Untreated Dry Cough

III. Home Remedies for Dry Cough
   A. Hydration and Moisture
   B. Herbal Teas and Infusions
   C. Honey and Lemon
   D. Steam Inhalation
   E. Gargling with Salt Water
   F. Throat Lozenges and Pastilles
   G. Use of Humidifiers
   H. Breathing Exercises

IV. Over-the-Counter Medications
   A. Antitussives
   B. Expectorants
   C. Decongestants

    D. Analgesics and NSAIDs

V. Natural Supplements and Herbs
    A. Echinacea
    B. Ginger
    C. Marshmallow Root
    D. Slippery Elm
    E. Licorice Root

VI. Lifestyle and Dietary Considerations
    A. Avoiding Irritants
    B. Dietary Modifications
    C. Proper Sleep Hygiene

VII. Professional Medical Treatment Options
    A. Prescription Medications
    B. Immunotherapy
    C. Referral to a Specialist

VIII. Prevention Strategies
    A. Hand Hygiene
    B. Vaccinations
    C. Avoiding Exposure to Allergens and Irritants

IX. When to Seek Medical Attention
    A. Persistent or Severe Symptoms
    B. Complications Associated with Dry Cough
    C. Underlying Health Conditions

X. **Conclusion**
   A. Summary of Key Points
   B. Encouragement for Seeking Appropriate Treatment

Chapter 1

I. Introduction to Dry Cough

A dry cough is a type of cough that does not produce any mucus or phlegm. It is often characterized by a tickling sensation or irritation in the throat, leading to repetitive coughing without bringing up any secretions. While it may not be as severe as a productive cough, a dry cough can still be bothersome and may interfere with daily activities and sleep.

A. **Definition and Characteristics**
   1. Definition of Dry Cough
   2. Differentiating Dry Cough from Productive Cough

B. **Causes of Dry Cough**
   1. Common Causes:
      a. Viral Infections (e.g., common cold, flu)
      b. Allergies (e.g., hay fever, dust mites, pet dander)
      c. Environmental Irritants (e.g., smoke, pollution)
      d. Asthma
      e. Postnasal Drip
   2. Less Common Causes:

a. Gastroesophageal Reflux Disease (GERD)
   b. Medications (e.g., ACE inhibitors)
   c. Chronic Respiratory Conditions (e.g., COPD)
   d. Lung Infections (e.g., pneumonia)
   e. Pertussis (Whooping Cough)

C. **Common Symptoms Associated with Dry Cough**
   1. Tickling Sensation in Throat
   2. Persistent or Intermittent Coughing
   3. Sore Throat
   4. Hoarseness
   5. Difficulty Breathing (in severe cases)

Understanding these introductory aspects of dry cough sets the stage for exploring its treatment and management strategies.

A. **Definition and Characteristics**

1. **Definition of Dry Cough**:
   - A dry cough, also known as a non-productive cough, is a cough that does not produce any phlegm or mucus.
   - It is characterized by the absence of secretions in the airways, leading to a persistent, often irritating coughing reflex.

2. **Differentiating Dry Cough from Productive Cough**:
   - Dry cough: Produces no mucus or phlegm, often accompanied by a tickling sensation in the throat.
   - Productive cough: Produces mucus or phlegm, which may vary in color and consistency, aiding in clearing the airways.

Understanding the distinction between dry cough and productive cough helps in identifying the appropriate treatment and management strategies tailored to the underlying cause.

B. **Causes of Dry Cough**

1. **Common Causes**:
   a. **Viral Infections**:
      - Common cold
      - Influenza (flu)
      - Respiratory syncytial virus (RSV) infection
   b. **Allergies**:
      - Hay fever (allergic rhinitis)
      - Allergic reactions to dust mites, pollen, mold, or pet dander
   c. **Environmental Irritants**:
      - Tobacco smoke
      - Air pollution

- Chemical fumes or irritants
  d. **Asthma**:
   - Allergic asthma
   - Exercise-induced asthma
   - Occupational asthma
  e. **Postnasal Drip**:
   - Sinus infections (sinusitis)
   - Rhinitis (inflammation of the nasal passages)
   - Nasal polyps

2. **Less Common Causes**:
  a. **Gastroesophageal Reflux Disease (GERD)**:
   - Acid reflux irritates the throat, leading to a dry cough.
  b. **Medications**:
   - Angiotensin-converting enzyme (ACE) inhibitors can cause a persistent dry cough in some individuals.
  c. **Chronic Respiratory Conditions**:
   - Chronic obstructive pulmonary disease (COPD)
   - Bronchiectasis
   - Interstitial lung diseases
  d. **Lung Infections**:
   - Pneumonia
   - Tuberculosis (TB)
   - Fungal infections

e. **Pertussis (Whooping Cough)**:
   - A bacterial infection causing severe bouts of coughing, often with a characteristic "whooping" sound.

Identifying the underlying cause of dry cough is crucial for effective treatment and management. In some cases, medical evaluation may be necessary to determine the specific cause.

C. Common Symptoms Associated with Dry Cough

1. **Tickling Sensation in Throat**:
   - Individuals with a dry cough often experience a persistent tickling or irritation sensation in the throat, triggering the cough reflex.

2. **Persistent or Intermittent Coughing**:
   - Dry coughs can be characterized by repetitive, non-productive coughing spells that occur throughout the day or night.

3. **Sore Throat**:
   - The continuous coughing associated with a dry cough can lead to throat discomfort and soreness.

4. **Hoarseness**:
   - Prolonged coughing episodes may result in hoarseness or changes in voice quality due to strain on the vocal cords.

5. **Difficulty Breathing (in severe cases)**:
   - In some instances, especially if the underlying cause is asthma or another respiratory condition, individuals may experience difficulty breathing or shortness of breath during or after coughing fits.

6. **Sleep Disturbances**:
   - Dry coughs can disrupt sleep patterns, leading to insomnia or poor sleep quality due to frequent nighttime coughing episodes.

7. **Fatigue and Irritability**:
   - Chronic dry coughing can contribute to fatigue and irritability due to the physical strain and lack of restful sleep.

8. **Limited Physical Activity**:
   - Severe or persistent dry coughs may limit individuals' ability to engage in physical activities or perform daily tasks comfortably.

Recognizing these common symptoms associated with dry coughs can help individuals seek appropriate treatment and management strategies to alleviate discomfort and improve quality of life.

Chapter 2

Understanding the Importance of Treating Dry Cough

A dry cough, although often considered less severe than a productive cough, can have significant implications for an individual's health and well-being. Addressing and treating dry coughs promptly is essential to prevent potential complications and improve overall quality of life.

A. **Impact on Quality of Life**
1. **Disruption of Daily Activities**: Persistent coughing spells can interfere with work, school, and other daily responsibilities, leading to decreased productivity and performance.
2. **Sleep Disturbances**: Nighttime coughing can disrupt sleep patterns, causing insomnia, fatigue, and daytime drowsiness.
3. **Physical Discomfort**: The constant irritation and strain on the throat caused by dry coughing can result in soreness, hoarseness, and overall physical discomfort.
4. **Psychological Effects**: Chronic coughing may lead to frustration, anxiety, and decreased self-esteem, impacting mental well-being and overall quality of life.

B. Potential Complications of Untreated Dry Cough

1. **Respiratory Infections**: Prolonged coughing weakens the immune system and increases susceptibility to respiratory infections such as bronchitis and pneumonia.
2. **Musculoskeletal Strain**: Persistent coughing can strain the muscles of the chest, abdomen, and back, leading to pain and discomfort.
3. **Worsening Underlying Conditions**: Ignoring a dry cough may allow underlying conditions such as asthma or GERD to worsen over time, potentially leading to more severe symptoms and complications.
4. **Sleep Disorders**: Chronic coughing can contribute to the development of sleep disorders such as insomnia and sleep apnea, further exacerbating fatigue and daytime sleepiness.
5. **Social Isolation**: Embarrassment or discomfort associated with frequent coughing may lead to social withdrawal and isolation, affecting relationships and mental well-being.

Understanding the importance of treating dry coughs goes beyond symptom management; it involves addressing underlying causes, preventing complications, and improving overall quality of life. Prompt intervention and appropriate management strategies are key to mitigating the impact of dry coughs on physical and emotional health.

A. Impact on Quality of Life

1. Disruption of Daily Activities:
- Persistent coughing spells can disrupt daily routines, making it challenging to focus on work, school, or household chores.
- Individuals may feel compelled to limit social interactions or avoid public spaces due to embarrassment or discomfort associated with frequent coughing.

2. Sleep Disturbances:
- Nighttime coughing episodes can significantly impair sleep quality, leading to insomnia, frequent awakenings, and daytime fatigue.
- Chronic sleep disturbances may contribute to mood disturbances, irritability, and decreased cognitive function during waking hours.

3. Physical Discomfort:
- The constant irritation and strain on the throat and chest muscles can cause soreness, hoarseness, and discomfort.

- Prolonged coughing may lead to headaches, chest pain, and abdominal muscle strain, further affecting comfort and well-being.

4. **Psychological Effects**:
   - Living with a chronic dry cough can take a toll on mental health, leading to increased stress, anxiety, and frustration.
   - Individuals may experience feelings of embarrassment, self-consciousness, or social isolation, impacting self-esteem and overall emotional well-being.

5. **Decreased Productivity and Engagement**:
   - The physical and emotional burden of dealing with a persistent cough can diminish productivity and engagement in activities.
   - Individuals may struggle to concentrate, complete tasks efficiently, or participate in recreational activities they enjoy.

6. **Limitations in Physical Activity**:
   - Severe coughing spells may limit individuals' ability to engage in physical exercise or activities, leading to decreased fitness levels and potential weight gain.

- Avoidance of physical exertion due to fear of triggering coughing fits can further contribute to a sedentary lifestyle and its associated health risks.

7. **Impact on Relationships**:
  - Chronic coughing can strain relationships with family, friends, and colleagues, especially if others perceive it as disruptive or bothersome.
  - Individuals may feel isolated or misunderstood, leading to communication barriers and interpersonal challenges.

Addressing the impact of dry cough on quality of life involves not only managing the physical symptoms but also providing support for the emotional and social aspects of living with a chronic condition. Effective treatment and coping strategies can help minimize disruptions and improve overall well-being for individuals affected by dry cough.

B. **Potential Complications of Untreated Dry Cough**

1. **Respiratory Infections**:
  - Persistent coughing weakens the respiratory defenses, increasing the risk of developing

secondary bacterial or viral infections such as bronchitis or pneumonia.
 - These infections can be more severe and require additional medical intervention, including antibiotics or antiviral medications.

2. **Musculoskeletal Strain**:
 - Chronic coughing can strain the muscles of the chest, abdomen, and back, leading to discomfort, pain, and even musculoskeletal injuries.
 - Over time, this strain may contribute to persistent soreness, reduced mobility, and decreased quality of life.

3. **Worsening Underlying Conditions**:
 - Ignoring a dry cough may allow underlying medical conditions such as asthma, chronic obstructive pulmonary disease (COPD), or gastroesophageal reflux disease (GERD) to worsen.
 - Untreated underlying conditions can lead to progressive respiratory impairment, exacerbations of symptoms, and complications requiring more aggressive treatment.

4. **Sleep Disorders**:
 - Chronic coughing can disrupt normal sleep patterns, leading to sleep disturbances such as insomnia, fragmented sleep, and daytime fatigue.

- Prolonged sleep disruption may impair cognitive function, mood regulation, and overall quality of life, increasing the risk of developing sleep disorders such as sleep apnea.

5. **Social Isolation**:
   - Embarrassment, discomfort, or inconvenience associated with frequent coughing may lead to social withdrawal, avoidance of social gatherings, or reluctance to engage in public activities.
   - Social isolation can negatively impact mental health, leading to feelings of loneliness, depression, and anxiety, further exacerbating the effects of untreated coughing.

6. **Compromised Immune Function**:
   - Chronic coughing can place additional stress on the immune system, potentially compromising its ability to defend against infections and other illnesses.
   - Reduced immune function may lead to more frequent illnesses, longer recovery times, and increased susceptibility to complications.

7. **Decreased Quality of Life**:
   - Left untreated, chronic dry cough can significantly impair quality of life, affecting physical

health, emotional well-being, and social functioning.

   - The cumulative effects of untreated coughing can lead to functional limitations, reduced independence, and diminished overall satisfaction with life.

Addressing and treating dry cough promptly is essential to minimize the risk of complications, improve symptoms, and enhance overall well-being. Seeking medical evaluation and adopting appropriate management strategies can help prevent long-term consequences associated with untreated coughing.

Chapter 3

Home Remedies for Dry Cough

Home remedies can often provide relief from dry cough symptoms and help soothe the throat. These natural remedies are generally safe and can be easily incorporated into daily routines for symptom management.

A. **Hydration and Moisture**

1. Drinking plenty of fluids, such as water, herbal teas, or warm broth, helps keep the throat hydrated and soothes irritation.
2. Using a humidifier or steam inhalation can add moisture to the air, reducing throat dryness and easing coughing.

B. **Herbal Teas and Infusions**

1. Herbal teas containing ingredients like ginger, chamomile, peppermint, or licorice root can provide soothing relief for dry coughs.
2. Adding honey or lemon to herbal teas may enhance their soothing properties and help alleviate throat irritation.

C. **Honey and Lemon**

1. Consuming a teaspoon of honey or lemon mixed with warm water can help coat the throat and reduce coughing.

2. Honey has natural antimicrobial properties, while lemon provides vitamin C and antioxidants to support immune health.

D. **Steam Inhalation**

1. Inhaling steam from a bowl of hot water or a steamy shower can help moisten the airways, loosen mucus, and ease dry cough symptoms.

2. Adding essential oils such as eucalyptus or peppermint to the steam can provide additional respiratory relief.

E. **Gargling with Salt Water**

1. Gargling with warm salt water helps reduce throat inflammation, soothe irritation, and alleviate dry cough symptoms.

2. Mix one-half to one teaspoon of salt in a glass of warm water and gargle for 30 seconds before spitting it out.

F. **Throat Lozenges and Pastilles**

1. Sucking on throat lozenges or pastilles containing menthol, eucalyptus, or honey can help

soothe throat irritation and suppress cough reflexes.

2. Choose lozenges without sugar or artificial additives for optimal throat comfort.

G. **Use of Humidifiers**

1. Using a humidifier in the bedroom or other commonly used areas helps maintain optimal humidity levels, preventing throat dryness and reducing coughing.

2. Clean humidifiers regularly to prevent bacterial growth and maintain air quality.

H. **Breathing Exercises**

1. Practicing deep breathing exercises, such as diaphragmatic breathing or pursed-lip breathing, can help relax the respiratory muscles and reduce coughing.

2. Breathing exercises also promote better lung function and oxygenation, supporting overall respiratory health.

These home remedies offer natural and accessible ways to alleviate dry cough symptoms and promote throat comfort. However, individuals with persistent or severe cough symptoms should consult a healthcare professional for proper diagnosis and treatment.

A. **Hydration and Moisture**

1. **Drinking Plenty of Fluids**:
   - Adequate hydration is essential for maintaining moisture in the throat and respiratory tract, reducing throat irritation, and soothing dry cough.
   - Recommended fluids include water, herbal teas, warm broth, and clear soups.
   - Avoiding caffeinated and alcoholic beverages, as they can contribute to dehydration.

2. **Using a Humidifier**:
   - Adding moisture to the air with a humidifier can help alleviate dry cough by preventing dryness in the throat and airways.
   - Place a humidifier in the bedroom or commonly used areas, especially during dry weather or winter months when indoor air tends to be drier.
   - Clean the humidifier regularly to prevent the growth of mold and bacteria, which can worsen respiratory symptoms.

3. **Steam Inhalation**:
   - Inhaling steam from a bowl of hot water or a steamy shower can provide immediate relief for dry cough.

- Steam helps moisturize the throat, loosen mucus, and ease coughing by soothing irritated airways.
   - Adding essential oils such as eucalyptus or peppermint to the steam can provide additional respiratory benefits.

4. **Avoiding Dehydrating Substances**:
   - Limiting consumption of dehydrating substances like caffeine and alcohol can help maintain optimal hydration levels and prevent exacerbation of dry cough symptoms.
   - These substances can contribute to dryness in the throat and exacerbate coughing, so it's best to minimize their intake, especially during periods of coughing.

Ensuring adequate hydration and moisture in the throat and airways is a fundamental aspect of managing dry cough symptoms. Incorporating these simple strategies into daily routines can help alleviate discomfort and promote respiratory health.

B. Herbal Teas and Infusions

1. Ginger Tea:
- Ginger has anti-inflammatory and antimicrobial properties that can help soothe throat irritation and reduce coughing.
- Steep fresh ginger slices or grated ginger root in hot water for 5-10 minutes, then strain and drink.
- Adding honey and lemon to ginger tea can enhance its flavor and therapeutic benefits.

2. Chamomile Tea:
- Chamomile has calming and anti-inflammatory properties, making it effective for soothing throat discomfort and reducing coughing.
- Steep chamomile tea bags or dried chamomile flowers in hot water for 5-10 minutes, then strain and enjoy.
- Chamomile tea is particularly beneficial for promoting relaxation and improving sleep quality.

3. Peppermint Tea:
- Peppermint contains menthol, which acts as a natural decongestant and throat relaxant, helping to relieve coughing and ease breathing.
- Steep peppermint tea bags or fresh peppermint leaves in hot water for 5-10 minutes, then strain and drink.

- Peppermint tea has a refreshing flavor and can help clear nasal passages and soothe throat irritation.

4. **Licorice Root Tea**:
   - Licorice root has demulcent properties, meaning it forms a soothing film over the throat lining, reducing irritation and coughing.
   - Steep licorice root tea bags or dried licorice root slices in hot water for 5-10 minutes, then strain and enjoy.
   - Licorice root tea has a sweet and slightly earthy flavor, making it a popular choice for soothing dry cough symptoms.

5. **Thyme Tea**:
   - Thyme contains compounds with expectorant and antimicrobial properties that can help loosen mucus and relieve coughing.
   - Steep fresh or dried thyme leaves in hot water for 5-10 minutes, then strain and drink.
   - Thyme tea has a pleasant herbal flavor and can be enhanced with honey or lemon for added sweetness and throat soothing benefits.

Incorporating herbal teas and infusions into your daily routine can provide natural relief for dry cough symptoms while also offering additional health benefits. Experiment with different herbal blends and flavors to find the ones that work best for you.

C. Honey and Lemon

1. **Honey**:
   - Honey has natural antimicrobial and anti-inflammatory properties that can help soothe sore throat and suppress coughing.
   - It forms a protective coating over the throat, reducing irritation and providing relief from dry cough symptoms.
   - Consuming a teaspoon of raw honey alone or mixed with warm water can provide immediate relief for dry cough.

2. **Lemon**:
   - Lemon is rich in vitamin C and antioxidants, which support immune health and help fight off infections.
   - It also contains citric acid, which can help break up mucus and alleviate throat irritation.
   - Squeezing fresh lemon juice into warm water or herbal tea and adding honey to taste creates a soothing and refreshing drink for dry cough relief.

3. **Honey and Lemon Drink**:
   - Combining honey and lemon creates a powerful natural remedy for dry cough.
   - Mix equal parts of honey and freshly squeezed lemon juice in warm water, stirring until well combined.
   - Sip on this soothing drink throughout the day to moisturize the throat, suppress coughing, and boost immune function.

4. **Honey-Lemon Cough Syrup**:
   - To make a homemade cough syrup, mix together equal parts of honey and lemon juice in a small container.
   - Take one to two teaspoons of the syrup as needed to relieve dry cough symptoms.
   - Store the syrup in the refrigerator for up to one week and shake well before each use.

5. **Precautions**:
   - Note that honey should not be given to infants under one year of age due to the risk of infant botulism.
   - Use caution when consuming lemon juice if you have sensitive teeth or acid reflux, as it may exacerbate these conditions in some individuals.

Incorporating honey and lemon into your daily routine can provide natural relief for dry cough symptoms while also supporting overall health and well-being. Adjust the ratio of honey to lemon according to your taste preferences and symptom severity.

D. **Steam Inhalation**

1. **Method**:
   - Boil water in a pot or kettle until it produces steam.
   - Carefully pour the hot water into a large bowl or basin.
   - Optional: Add a few drops of essential oils such as eucalyptus or peppermint to the water for added respiratory benefits.
   - Position your face over the bowl and drape a towel over your head to create a tent, trapping the steam.
   - Inhale deeply through your nose for several minutes, allowing the steam to penetrate your airways and soothe throat irritation.

2. **Benefits**:
   - Steam inhalation helps moisturize the respiratory passages, loosening mucus and phlegm and easing congestion.
   - It can also alleviate throat dryness and irritation, reducing coughing and promoting respiratory comfort.
   - Adding essential oils to the steam can provide additional therapeutic benefits, such as decongestion and relaxation.

3. **Precautions**:
   - Be cautious when handling hot water to avoid burns or scalds.
   - Keep a safe distance from the steam to prevent accidental injury.
   - Supervise children closely during steam inhalation to ensure their safety.
   - Individuals with certain respiratory conditions such as asthma should consult a healthcare professional before using steam inhalation, as it may exacerbate symptoms in some cases.

4. **Frequency**:
   - Steam inhalation can be performed several times a day or as needed to relieve dry cough symptoms.
   - It is particularly beneficial before bedtime to promote relaxation and improve sleep quality.

5. **Alternative Method**:
   - For a more convenient option, consider using a steam inhaler or facial steamer, which provides controlled steam delivery and may include additional features such as aromatherapy diffusion.

Steam inhalation is a simple yet effective home remedy for dry cough, providing immediate relief by moisturizing the airways and soothing throat irritation. Incorporate this natural remedy into your daily routine to alleviate coughing and promote respiratory comfort.

E. Gargling with Salt Water

1. **Preparation**:
   - Mix approximately half to one teaspoon of salt into a glass of warm water.
   - Stir the solution until the salt is completely dissolved.

2. **Gargling Technique**:
   - Take a sip of the saltwater solution and tilt your head back slightly.
   - Gargle the solution in your throat for about 30 seconds to one minute, allowing it to reach the back of your throat and the tonsils.

- Avoid swallowing the saltwater during gargling.
- Spit out the saltwater solution after gargling.

3. **Benefits**:
- Gargling with salt water helps to soothe throat irritation and reduce inflammation, providing relief from dry cough.
- The saltwater solution helps to draw out excess mucus and bacteria from the throat, promoting a cleaner and healthier environment.
- Salt has antiseptic properties that can help kill bacteria and viruses in the throat, potentially reducing the risk of infection.

4. **Frequency**:
- Gargle with salt water several times a day or as needed to alleviate dry cough symptoms.
- It is particularly beneficial to gargle with salt water after meals or before bedtime to cleanse the throat and promote comfort.

5. **Precautions**:
- Avoid using excessive salt in the gargling solution, as it may cause irritation or discomfort.
- Do not swallow the saltwater solution, as it can lead to dehydration or electrolyte imbalance.
- Individuals with high blood pressure or other medical conditions should consult a healthcare

professional before using saltwater gargles regularly.

Gargling with salt water is a simple and effective home remedy for relieving dry cough symptoms and promoting throat comfort. Incorporate this natural remedy into your daily routine to soothe throat irritation and support respiratory health.

F. **Throat Lozenges and Pastilles**

1. **Selection**:
   - Choose throat lozenges or pastilles that contain soothing ingredients such as menthol, eucalyptus, honey, or herbal extracts.
   - Look for products labeled as sugar-free or with natural sweeteners to avoid excessive sugar intake.

2. **Usage**:
   - Place a throat lozenge or pastille in your mouth and allow it to dissolve slowly.
   - Suck on the lozenge or pastille periodically throughout the day or as needed to relieve throat irritation and suppress dry cough.
   - Avoid chewing or swallowing the lozenge whole, as it may diminish its effectiveness.

3. **Benefits**:
   - Throat lozenges and pastilles provide a soothing coating over the throat, reducing irritation and dryness.
   - Ingredients such as menthol or eucalyptus have a cooling effect that can help numb the throat and alleviate discomfort.
   - Some throat lozenges contain ingredients with mild anesthetic properties, providing temporary relief from sore throat and coughing.

4. **Varieties**:
   - Throat lozenges and pastilles come in various flavors and formulations to suit individual preferences.
   - Options include sugar-free varieties, herbal or natural formulations, and products with added vitamins or minerals for immune support.

5. **Precautions**:
   - Avoid giving throat lozenges or pastilles to young children, as they may pose a choking hazard.
   - Use throat lozenges and pastilles as directed and do not exceed the recommended dosage.
   - Some individuals may be allergic to certain ingredients in throat lozenges, so it's important to check the product label for potential allergens.

Throat lozenges and pastilles are convenient and portable remedies for dry cough symptoms, providing immediate relief and soothing throat irritation. Keep a supply of these throat-soothing products on hand for quick and effective relief throughout the day.

G. **Use of Humidifiers**

1. **Selection**:
   - Choose a humidifier that suits your needs and preferences, such as a cool mist or warm mist humidifier.
   - Consider the size of the room where the humidifier will be used to ensure adequate coverage.
   - Look for features such as adjustable humidity settings, timers, and automatic shut-off for convenience and ease of use.

2. **Placement**:
   - Position the humidifier in the bedroom or other commonly used areas where you spend the most time.
   - Place the humidifier on a flat, stable surface away from direct sunlight and heat sources.

- Keep the humidifier at least a few feet away from walls and furniture to allow for proper airflow and moisture distribution.

3. **Operation**:
  - Fill the humidifier's water tank with clean, filtered water according to the manufacturer's instructions.
  - Adjust the humidity settings to achieve the desired level of moisture in the air.
  - Run the humidifier continuously or as needed, especially during dry weather or winter months when indoor air tends to be drier.
  - Clean the humidifier regularly to prevent the buildup of mold, bacteria, and mineral deposits, following the manufacturer's instructions for maintenance.

4. **Benefits**:
  - Humidifiers add moisture to the air, helping to alleviate dryness in the throat and respiratory tract.
  - Increased humidity can soothe throat irritation, reduce coughing, and promote respiratory comfort, especially for individuals with dry cough symptoms.
  - Humidifiers can also improve indoor air quality by reducing dust, allergens, and airborne pollutants, creating a healthier environment for breathing.

5. **Precautions**:
   - Monitor humidity levels regularly to prevent excessive moisture buildup, which can promote mold growth and other respiratory issues.
   - Use distilled or demineralized water in the humidifier to minimize the risk of mineral deposits and microbial contamination.
   - Clean and maintain the humidifier according to the manufacturer's instructions to ensure optimal performance and safety.

Incorporating a humidifier into your home environment can provide numerous benefits for respiratory health and alleviate symptoms of dry cough. Use a humidifier regularly to maintain optimal humidity levels and promote comfort and well-being.

H. **Breathing Exercises**

1. **Diaphragmatic Breathing (Deep Breathing)**:
   - Sit or lie down in a comfortable position with your back straight.
   - Place one hand on your chest and the other on your abdomen.

- Inhale deeply through your nose, allowing your abdomen to rise as you fill your lungs with air.
- Exhale slowly and fully through your mouth, feeling your abdomen fall as you release the air.
- Repeat this deep breathing pattern for several minutes, focusing on relaxing your body and calming your mind.

2. **Pursed-Lip Breathing**:
- Sit or stand in a relaxed position with your back straight.
- Inhale slowly and deeply through your nose for a count of two.
- Purse your lips as if you were going to whistle or blow out a candle.
- Exhale slowly and gently through pursed lips for a count of four, allowing the exhale to be twice as long as the inhale.
- Repeat this pursed-lip breathing pattern for several breaths, focusing on maintaining a steady and controlled breath flow.

3. **Alternate Nostril Breathing (Nadi Shodhana)**:
- Sit comfortably with your spine straight and shoulders relaxed.
- Place your left hand on your left knee with the palm facing up.

- Use your right hand to close your right nostril with your thumb and inhale deeply through your left nostril.
- Release your right nostril and close your left nostril with your ring finger, exhaling slowly through your right nostril.
- Inhale through your right nostril, then close it with your thumb and exhale through your left nostril.
- Continue alternating between inhaling and exhaling through each nostril, focusing on smooth and controlled breathing.

4. **Box Breathing (Square Breathing)**:
- Sit or stand in a comfortable position with your back straight.
- Inhale deeply through your nose for a count of four, imagining you are tracing the first side of a square.
- Hold your breath for a count of four, visualizing the second side of the square.
- Exhale slowly and completely through your mouth for a count of four, tracing the third side of the square.
- Hold your breath again for a count of four, completing the square.
- Repeat this box breathing pattern for several cycles, focusing on relaxation and stress reduction.

Breathing exercises can help improve lung function, reduce stress, and promote relaxation, making them valuable tools for managing dry cough symptoms. Incorporate these simple exercises into your daily routine to enhance respiratory health and overall well-being.

Chapter 4

Over-the-Counter Medications

While home remedies and lifestyle modifications can often provide relief for dry cough, over-the-counter (OTC) medications can be useful for managing persistent symptoms or addressing underlying causes. It's important to choose OTC medications carefully and use them according to the manufacturer's instructions or a healthcare professional's recommendation.

A. **Cough Suppressants**:
  1. **Dextromethorphan (DM)**:
   - Suppresses cough reflex by acting on the cough center in the brain.
   - Available in various forms, including syrups, lozenges, and tablets.
   - Use caution when combining with other medications, as it may interact with certain drugs or cause drowsiness.
  2. **Codeine (available in some formulations)**:
   - Suppresses cough reflex by acting on the central nervous system.

- Typically available in combination with other medications, such as acetaminophen or guaifenesin.
- Requires a prescription in some countries due to its potential for abuse and dependence.

B. **Expectorants**:
  - **Guaifenesin**:
    - Helps loosen and thin mucus in the airways, making it easier to expel through coughing.
    - Available in various formulations, including syrups, tablets, and extended-release tablets.
    - Drink plenty of fluids while taking guaifenesin to enhance its effectiveness in thinning mucus.

C. **Decongestants**:
  - **Pseudoephedrine**:
    - Relieves nasal congestion by constricting blood vessels in the nasal passages.
    - Available in tablet or liquid form, often combined with other cold or flu medications.
    - Use caution in individuals with certain medical conditions, such as high blood pressure or heart disease.
  - **Phenylephrine**:
    - Acts similarly to pseudoephedrine but is less effective and may have fewer side effects.
    - Available in nasal spray or oral tablet form.

D. **Antihistamines**:
   - **Diphenhydramine (Benadryl)**:
      - Helps relieve allergy symptoms such as sneezing, runny nose, and itchy throat, which may contribute to coughing.
      - Can cause drowsiness, so it is often taken at bedtime.
   - **Loratadine (Claritin) or cetirizine (Zyrtec)**:
      - Non-drowsy antihistamines that provide relief from allergy symptoms without causing significant sedation.

E. **Nasal Sprays**:
   - **Saline Nasal Spray**:
      - Helps moisturize nasal passages and relieve nasal congestion.
      - Safe for use in adults and children, and can be used as often as needed.

Before using any OTC medication, it's important to read the label carefully and follow the recommended dosage instructions. If you have any questions or concerns about OTC medications, consult with a pharmacist or healthcare professional for guidance tailored to your specific needs and medical history.

A. **Antitussives**

Antitussives are medications specifically designed to suppress coughing by acting on the cough reflex. They can be useful for providing relief from dry, non-productive cough associated with conditions such as colds, flu, or irritants. Here are some common antitussive medications:

1. **Dextromethorphan (DM)**:
   - Dextromethorphan is one of the most commonly used antitussive medications available over the counter.
   - It works by suppressing the cough reflex in the brain, providing relief from coughing.
   - Available in various forms including syrups, lozenges, and capsules.
   - It's important to use dextromethorphan as directed and to avoid exceeding the recommended dosage, as misuse can lead to adverse effects such as dizziness, drowsiness, or even overdose.

2. **Codeine**:
   - Codeine is a stronger antitussive medication that is sometimes used to treat severe or persistent coughing.
   - It works by suppressing coughing through its effects on the central nervous system.

- Codeine-containing medications are available in some countries, often combined with other ingredients such as acetaminophen or guaifenesin.
- Due to its potential for abuse and dependence, codeine is typically available by prescription only in many regions.

3. **Benzonatate**:
- Benzonatate is a non-narcotic antitussive medication that works by numbing the throat and lungs, reducing the urge to cough.
- It is available in capsule form and should be swallowed whole, as chewing or dissolving the capsules can lead to adverse effects such as numbing of the mouth and throat.
- Benzonatate is available over the counter in some countries, but it may require a prescription in others.

4. **Pholcodine**:
- Pholcodine is another antitussive medication that works by suppressing the cough reflex in the brain.
- It is available in some countries and may be found in cough syrups or lozenges.
- Like other antitussives, pholcodine should be used according to the recommended dosage and precautions to avoid adverse effects.

It's important to note that while antitussive medications can provide relief from coughing, they do not treat the underlying cause of the cough. If cough symptoms persist or worsen despite treatment with antitussives, it's advisable to consult a healthcare professional for further evaluation and management. Additionally, certain populations such as children, pregnant or breastfeeding individuals, and those with certain medical conditions may need to exercise caution or seek medical advice before using antitussive medications.

B. Expectorants

Expectorants are medications that help loosen and thin mucus in the respiratory tract, making it easier to cough up and expel. They are commonly used to relieve symptoms of chest congestion and productive cough associated with respiratory infections or conditions such as bronchitis or pneumonia. Here are some common expectorant medications:

1. **Guaifenesin**:
   - Guaifenesin is one of the most widely used expectorant medications available over the counter.

- It works by increasing the volume and reducing the viscosity of respiratory tract secretions, making them easier to clear.
- Guaifenesin is available in various formulations including syrups, tablets, and extended-release tablets.
- It is generally well-tolerated, but side effects may include gastrointestinal upset, dizziness, or drowsiness in some individuals.

2. **Bromhexine**:
- Bromhexine is another expectorant medication that works by increasing the production of respiratory tract secretions and reducing their viscosity.
- It is available in some countries and may be found in cough syrups or tablets.
- Bromhexine is often used to relieve symptoms of acute respiratory conditions such as bronchitis or pneumonia.

3. **Ipecacuanha**:
- Ipecacuanha is a natural expectorant derived from the root of the ipecac plant.
- It works by stimulating the bronchial glands to increase mucus production and promote coughing.

- Ipecacuanha is available in some herbal cough remedies and may be used to relieve chest congestion and productive cough.

4. **Ammonium Chloride**:
   - Ammonium chloride is an expectorant medication that works by irritating the respiratory tract lining, leading to increased mucus production and coughing.
   - It is available in some cough syrups or lozenges and may be used to relieve symptoms of chest congestion and productive cough.

Expectorant medications can be helpful for individuals experiencing chest congestion and productive cough associated with respiratory illnesses. However, it's important to use expectorants as directed and to consult a healthcare professional if symptoms persist or worsen. Additionally, certain populations such as children, pregnant or breastfeeding individuals, and those with certain medical conditions may need to exercise caution or seek medical advice before using expectorant medications.

C. Decongestants

Decongestants are medications commonly used to relieve nasal congestion and sinus pressure associated with upper respiratory infections, allergies, or sinusitis. They work by narrowing blood vessels in the nasal passages, reducing swelling and congestion. Here are some common decongestant medications:

1. **Pseudoephedrine**:
   - Pseudoephedrine is a widely used decongestant available in oral tablet or liquid form.
   - It works by stimulating alpha-adrenergic receptors in the nasal mucosa, causing vasoconstriction and reducing nasal congestion.
   - Pseudoephedrine is often found in combination with other cold or allergy medications and may be available over the counter or behind the pharmacy counter, depending on local regulations.
   - It is important to use pseudoephedrine as directed and to avoid exceeding the recommended dosage, as misuse can lead to adverse effects such as increased heart rate, elevated blood pressure, or insomnia.

2. **Phenylephrine**:
   - Phenylephrine is a decongestant medication similar to pseudoephedrine, but it is less effective and has a shorter duration of action.
   - It is often found in nasal spray or oral tablet form and may be used to relieve nasal congestion associated with colds, allergies, or sinusitis.
   - Phenylephrine is generally well-tolerated, but it may cause side effects such as nervousness, dizziness, or increased blood pressure in some individuals.

3. **Oxymetazoline**:
   - Oxymetazoline is a topical decongestant available in nasal spray form.
   - It works by constricting blood vessels in the nasal passages, providing rapid relief from nasal congestion.
   - Oxymetazoline nasal spray is commonly used for short-term relief of nasal congestion due to colds, allergies, or sinusitis.
   - It is important to use oxymetazoline nasal spray as directed and to avoid prolonged or excessive use, as it may lead to rebound congestion or nasal irritation.

4. **Xylometazoline**:
   - Xylometazoline is another topical decongestant available in nasal spray form.
   - It works by constricting blood vessels in the nasal mucosa, reducing nasal congestion and sinus pressure.
   - Xylometazoline nasal spray is commonly used for short-term relief of nasal congestion associated with colds, allergies, or sinusitis.
   - Like oxymetazoline, it is important to use xylometazoline nasal spray as directed and to avoid prolonged or excessive use to prevent rebound congestion or nasal irritation.

Decongestant medications can provide effective relief from nasal congestion and sinus pressure, but they should be used judiciously and according to the manufacturer's instructions to minimize the risk of adverse effects. Individuals with certain medical conditions such as high blood pressure, heart disease, or thyroid disorders should consult a healthcare professional before using decongestant medications. Additionally, decongestants may interact with other medications, so it's important to check for potential drug interactions before use.

D. **Analgesics and NSAIDs (Nonsteroidal Anti-Inflammatory Drugs)**

Analgesics and NSAIDs are commonly used to relieve pain and reduce inflammation associated with various conditions, including respiratory infections, headaches, and muscle aches. While they do not directly treat the underlying cause of cough, they can help alleviate discomfort and improve overall well-being. Here are some common analgesics and NSAIDs:

1. **Acetaminophen (Tylenol):**
   - Acetaminophen is a widely used analgesic and antipyretic medication that is effective for relieving pain and reducing fever.
   - It works by inhibiting the production of prostaglandins in the brain, which are involved in pain perception and fever regulation.
   - Acetaminophen is available in various formulations including tablets, capsules, and liquid suspensions, and it is generally well-tolerated when used as directed.
   - It is important to avoid exceeding the recommended dosage of acetaminophen, as overdose can cause liver damage.

2. **Ibuprofen (Advil, Motrin) and Naproxen (Aleve):**
   - Ibuprofen and naproxen are NSAIDs that work by inhibiting the production of prostaglandins, which are involved in inflammation, pain, and fever.
   - They are commonly used to relieve mild to moderate pain associated with conditions such as headaches, muscle aches, and menstrual cramps.
   - Ibuprofen and naproxen are available in tablet, capsule, and liquid form, and they are generally well-tolerated when used as directed.
   - Side effects of NSAIDs may include gastrointestinal upset, stomach ulcers, and an increased risk of cardiovascular events, especially with long-term use or at high doses.

3. **Aspirin (Bayer, Bufferin):**
   - Aspirin is an NSAID that is commonly used to relieve pain, reduce inflammation, and prevent blood clotting.
   - It works by inhibiting the production of prostaglandins and thromboxanes, which are involved in pain, inflammation, and blood clotting.
   - Aspirin is available in various formulations including tablets, chewable tablets, and enteric-coated tablets.

- While aspirin is generally well-tolerated when used as directed, it may cause gastrointestinal upset, stomach ulcers, and an increased risk of bleeding, especially at high doses.

4. **Combination Products**:
   - Some over-the-counter cough and cold medications may contain a combination of analgesics, NSAIDs, decongestants, antihistamines, and/or cough suppressants.
   - These combination products are designed to provide relief from multiple symptoms associated with respiratory infections or allergies.
   - It is important to carefully read the label of combination products and to avoid taking multiple medications that contain the same active ingredients to prevent accidental overdose.

Before using analgesics or NSAIDs, it is important to read the label carefully and to use them as directed. Individuals with certain medical conditions such as liver disease, kidney disease, or gastrointestinal ulcers should consult a healthcare professional before using these medications. Additionally, NSAIDs may interact with other medications, so it is important to check for potential drug interactions before use. If pain or discomfort persists despite treatment with analgesics or NSAIDs, it is advisable to consult a healthcare professional for further evaluation and management.

Chapter 5

Natural Supplements and Herbs

Natural supplements and herbs can be used as complementary approaches to help alleviate symptoms of dry cough and support overall respiratory health. While they may not directly treat the underlying cause of cough, they can provide relief from irritation and inflammation in the respiratory tract. Here are some common natural supplements and herbs used for managing dry cough:

1. **Honey**:
   - Honey has been used for centuries as a natural remedy for cough and throat irritation.
   - It has antimicrobial and soothing properties that can help alleviate dry cough and sore throat.
   - Honey can be taken alone or mixed with warm water, lemon, or herbal teas for added benefits.

2. **Ginger**:
   - Ginger has anti-inflammatory and antimicrobial properties that can help soothe throat irritation and reduce coughing.
   - It can be consumed fresh, as a tea, or in capsule form to provide relief from dry cough symptoms.

3. **Eucalyptus**:
   - Eucalyptus oil is commonly used as a natural decongestant and expectorant.
   - Inhaling eucalyptus steam or using eucalyptus oil in a diffuser can help relieve nasal congestion and promote easier breathing.

4. **Peppermint**:
   - Peppermint has menthol, which acts as a natural decongestant and throat relaxant, helping to relieve coughing and ease breathing.
   - Peppermint tea or inhaling peppermint steam can provide relief from dry cough symptoms.

5. **Licorice Root**:
   - Licorice root has demulcent properties, meaning it forms a soothing film over the throat lining, reducing irritation and coughing.
   - Licorice root tea or lozenges can be used to soothe dry cough and sore throat.

6. **Marshmallow Root**:
   - Marshmallow root contains mucilage, which forms a protective layer over the throat and soothes irritation.
   - Marshmallow root tea or capsules can help relieve dry cough and promote throat comfort.

7. **Thyme**:
   - Thyme contains compounds with expectorant and antimicrobial properties that can help loosen mucus and relieve coughing.
   - Thyme tea or inhaling thyme steam can provide relief from dry cough symptoms.

8. **Slippery Elm**:
   - Slippery elm contains mucilage, which forms a soothing coating over the throat and reduces irritation.
   - Slippery elm lozenges or capsules can help relieve dry cough and promote throat comfort.

Before using natural supplements and herbs, it is important to consult with a healthcare professional, especially if you have any underlying health conditions or are taking medications. Some natural remedies may interact with certain medications or may not be suitable for everyone. Additionally, it's important to use high-quality, reputable products and to follow dosage instructions carefully.

Echinacea

Echinacea is a popular herbal remedy that is commonly used to support immune function and alleviate symptoms of respiratory infections, including coughs, colds, and flu. It is derived from the Echinacea plant, which is native to North America and has been used for centuries by Native American tribes for its medicinal properties. Here are some key points about Echinacea:

1. **Immune Support**:
   - Echinacea is believed to stimulate the immune system by increasing the production of white blood cells, which play a key role in fighting off infections.
   - It contains active compounds such as alkamides, polysaccharides, and flavonoids, which have been shown to have immunomodulatory effects.

2. **Antiviral and Antibacterial Properties**:
   - Echinacea has been found to possess antiviral and antibacterial properties, which may help prevent and treat respiratory infections caused by viruses and bacteria.
   - It may help reduce the severity and duration of symptoms associated with respiratory infections, including cough, sore throat, and congestion.

3. **Anti-inflammatory Effects**:
   - Echinacea exhibits anti-inflammatory effects, which can help reduce inflammation in the

respiratory tract and alleviate symptoms of cough and congestion.

- It may help soothe irritated throat tissues and promote respiratory comfort.

4. **Forms and Dosage**:
   - Echinacea supplements are available in various forms, including capsules, tablets, liquid extracts, and teas.
   - Dosage recommendations may vary depending on the specific product and formulation.
   - It is important to follow the dosage instructions provided on the product label or to consult with a healthcare professional for personalized recommendations.

5. **Safety and Side Effects**:
   - Echinacea is generally considered safe for most people when used as directed.
   - Side effects are rare but may include gastrointestinal upset, allergic reactions, or skin rash in some individuals.
   - People with autoimmune disorders, allergies to plants in the Asteraceae family (such as ragweed, marigolds, or daisies), or certain medical conditions should consult with a healthcare professional before using Echinacea.

6. **Use as a Cough Remedy**:
   - Echinacea may be used as part of a holistic approach to managing cough symptoms associated with respiratory infections.
   - It can be taken orally as a supplement or consumed as a tea to support immune function and alleviate cough and cold symptoms.

Overall, Echinacea is a popular herbal remedy with potential benefits for supporting immune function and relieving symptoms of respiratory infections, including cough. However, more research is needed to fully understand its effectiveness and safety for cough relief. It is always advisable to consult with a healthcare professional before using Echinacea or any other herbal supplement, especially if you have any underlying health conditions or are taking medications.

Ginger

Ginger, known scientifically as Zingiber officinale, is a versatile herb that has been used for centuries in traditional medicine for its various health benefits. It is commonly used as a culinary spice as well as a natural remedy for a wide range of ailments, including coughs and respiratory issues.

Here are some key points about ginger and its potential benefits for managing cough:

1. **Anti-inflammatory Properties**:
   - Ginger contains bioactive compounds such as gingerol, which have potent anti-inflammatory effects.
   - These anti-inflammatory properties can help reduce inflammation in the respiratory tract, providing relief from cough and other respiratory symptoms.

2. **Antioxidant Effects**:
   - Ginger is rich in antioxidants, which help neutralize harmful free radicals in the body.
   - By reducing oxidative stress and inflammation, ginger may help alleviate symptoms of respiratory infections and support overall respiratory health.

3. **Mucolytic Action**:
   - Ginger has mucolytic properties, meaning it helps loosen and expel mucus from the respiratory tract.
   - This can be particularly beneficial for individuals experiencing chest congestion and productive coughs, as ginger may help clear excess mucus and improve breathing.

4. **Antitussive Effects**:
   - Some studies suggest that ginger may have antitussive effects, meaning it may help suppress coughing.
   - By soothing throat irritation and reducing the urge to cough, ginger can provide relief from dry cough symptoms.

5. **Immune Support**:
   - Ginger is known to have immune-boosting properties, which can help strengthen the body's natural defenses against respiratory infections.
   - Consuming ginger regularly may help support immune function and reduce the risk of developing coughs and colds.

6. **Ease of Use**:
   - Ginger can be consumed in various forms, including fresh ginger root, ginger tea, ginger capsules, or ginger supplements.
   - Ginger tea, in particular, is a popular and soothing remedy for cough and respiratory issues. Simply steep fresh ginger slices or ginger tea bags in hot water and drink it throughout the day.

7. **Safety and Precautions**:
   - Ginger is generally considered safe for most people when consumed in moderate amounts.

- However, some individuals may experience mild side effects such as heartburn, stomach upset, or allergic reactions.
- It is advisable to consult with a healthcare professional before using ginger supplements, especially if you have any underlying health conditions or are taking medications.

In summary, ginger is a natural remedy with potential benefits for managing cough symptoms and promoting respiratory health. Incorporating ginger into your diet or consuming ginger-based remedies may help alleviate coughing and support overall well-being. However, it's essential to use ginger safely and consult with a healthcare professional if you have any concerns or questions about its use for cough relief.

Marshmallow Root

Marshmallow root, also known as Althaea officinalis, is a herb with a long history of use in traditional medicine for its soothing and healing properties. It is commonly used to alleviate various respiratory issues, including coughs and sore throats. Here are some key points about marshmallow root and its potential benefits for managing cough:

1. **Demulcent Properties**:
   - Marshmallow root contains high levels of mucilage, a gel-like substance that forms a protective coating over the mucous membranes of the throat and respiratory tract.
   - This mucilaginous quality gives marshmallow root its demulcent properties, allowing it to soothe and lubricate irritated tissues, making it effective for relieving dry coughs and sore throats.

2. **Expectorant Action**:
   - While marshmallow root is primarily known for its demulcent properties, it also possesses mild expectorant effects.
   - By helping to loosen and expel mucus from the respiratory tract, marshmallow root can aid in relieving chest congestion and productive coughs.

3. **Anti-inflammatory Effects**:
   - Marshmallow root contains compounds with anti-inflammatory properties, which can help reduce inflammation in the throat and respiratory tract.

- This anti-inflammatory action may help alleviate cough symptoms by calming irritation and promoting healing.

4. **Immune Support**:
   - Marshmallow root contains antioxidants, which can help support immune function and protect against oxidative stress.
   - By bolstering the body's natural defenses, marshmallow root may help reduce the risk of developing coughs and respiratory infections.

5. **Ease of Use**:
   - Marshmallow root can be consumed in various forms, including teas, tinctures, capsules, and lozenges.
   - Marshmallow root tea, in particular, is a popular remedy for cough and sore throat. Simply steep dried marshmallow root in hot water for several minutes, then strain and drink the tea as needed.

6. **Safety and Precautions**:
   - Marshmallow root is generally considered safe for most people when used in appropriate doses.
   - However, individuals with certain medical conditions, such as diabetes or low blood sugar, should use caution when consuming marshmallow root, as it may affect blood sugar levels.

- Pregnant or breastfeeding individuals should consult with a healthcare professional before using marshmallow root.

In summary, marshmallow root is a natural remedy with mucilaginous and soothing properties that can help relieve coughs and sore throats. Incorporating marshmallow root into your diet or using marshmallow root-based remedies may provide relief from cough symptoms and support respiratory health. However, it's essential to use marshmallow root safely and consult with a healthcare professional if you have any concerns or questions about its use for cough relief.

Slippery Elm

Slippery elm, scientifically known as Ulmus rubra, is a tree native to North America that has been used for centuries in traditional medicine for its soothing and healing properties. Slippery elm bark is the part of the tree most commonly used for medicinal purposes. It contains mucilage, a gel-like substance that becomes slippery when mixed with water, giving it its name. Here are some key points about slippery elm and its potential benefits for managing cough:

1. **Demulcent Properties**:
   - Slippery elm bark is rich in mucilage, which gives it demulcent properties.
   - When consumed, slippery elm forms a soothing and protective coating over the mucous membranes of the throat and respiratory tract, helping to alleviate irritation and inflammation associated with coughs.

2. **Soothes Sore Throats**:
   - Slippery elm can help relieve sore throats by reducing inflammation and providing a soothing layer of protection.
   - It may also help reduce the urge to cough by calming irritated throat tissues.

3. **Mucolytic Action**:
   - In addition to its demulcent properties, slippery elm has mild mucolytic effects.
   - It can help loosen and thin mucus in the respiratory tract, making it easier to expel through coughing and reducing chest congestion.

4. **Anti-inflammatory Effects**:
   - Slippery elm contains compounds with anti-inflammatory properties, which can help reduce inflammation in the throat and respiratory tract.

- This anti-inflammatory action may further contribute to its effectiveness in relieving cough symptoms.

5. **Ease of Use**:
   - Slippery elm is commonly available in various forms, including teas, capsules, lozenges, and throat sprays.
   - Slippery elm tea, made by steeping powdered slippery elm bark in hot water, is a popular remedy for cough and sore throat. It can be consumed several times a day as needed for relief.

6. **Safety and Precautions**:
   - Slippery elm is generally considered safe for most people when used in appropriate doses.
   - However, individuals with certain medical conditions, such as diabetes or low blood sugar, should use caution when consuming slippery elm, as it may affect blood sugar levels.
   - Pregnant or breastfeeding individuals should consult with a healthcare professional before using slippery elm.

In summary, slippery elm is a natural remedy with demulcent, mucolytic, and anti-inflammatory properties that can help relieve coughs and sore throats. Incorporating slippery elm into your diet or using slippery elm-based remedies may provide relief from cough symptoms and support respiratory health. However, it's essential to use slippery elm safely and consult with a healthcare professional if you have any concerns or questions about its use for cough relief.

Licorice Root

Licorice root, derived from the Glycyrrhiza glabra plant, has been used for centuries in traditional medicine for its various health benefits. It is commonly used as a natural remedy for coughs, sore throats, and respiratory issues due to its soothing and anti-inflammatory properties. Here are some key points about licorice root and its potential benefits for managing cough:

1. **Demulcent Properties**:
    - Licorice root contains compounds that give it demulcent properties, allowing it to form a soothing and protective coating over the mucous membranes of the throat and respiratory tract.
    - This mucilaginous quality helps relieve irritation and inflammation, making it effective for soothing dry coughs and sore throats.

2. **Expectorant Action**:
   - Licorice root has expectorant effects, meaning it helps loosen and expel mucus from the respiratory tract.
   - By promoting the clearance of mucus, licorice root can help alleviate chest congestion and productive coughs.

3. **Anti-inflammatory Effects**:
   - Licorice root contains glycyrrhizin, a compound with potent anti-inflammatory properties.
   - These anti-inflammatory effects help reduce inflammation in the throat and respiratory tract, providing relief from cough symptoms.

4. **Antiviral and Antimicrobial Properties**:
   - Licorice root has been shown to possess antiviral and antimicrobial properties, which can help fight off respiratory infections.
   - By inhibiting the growth of viruses and bacteria, licorice root may help prevent and treat coughs and colds.

5. **Immune Support**:
   - Licorice root contains antioxidants, which help support immune function and protect against oxidative stress.

- By bolstering the body's natural defenses, licorice root may help reduce the severity and duration of coughs and respiratory infections.

6. **Ease of Use**:
   - Licorice root can be consumed in various forms, including teas, capsules, extracts, and lozenges.
   - Licorice root tea, made by steeping dried licorice root in hot water, is a popular remedy for cough and sore throat. It can be consumed several times a day as needed for relief.

7. **Safety and Precautions**:
   - While licorice root is generally considered safe for most people when consumed in moderate amounts, excessive or prolonged use may lead to side effects such as hypertension, hypokalemia (low potassium levels), and fluid retention.
   - Individuals with certain medical conditions, such as high blood pressure, heart disease, kidney disease, or diabetes, should use caution when consuming licorice root and may need to avoid it altogether.
   - Pregnant or breastfeeding individuals should consult with a healthcare professional before using licorice root.

In summary, licorice root is a natural remedy with demulcent, expectorant, anti-inflammatory, and immune-supporting properties that can help relieve coughs and sore throats. Incorporating licorice root into your diet or using licorice root-based remedies may provide relief from cough symptoms and support respiratory health. However, it's essential to use licorice root safely and consult with a healthcare professional if you have any concerns or questions about its use for cough relief.

Chapter 6

Lifestyle and Dietary Considerations

In addition to using remedies and supplements, certain lifestyle and dietary changes can help manage and alleviate dry cough. Here are some considerations:

1. **Hydration**:
   - Drink plenty of fluids, such as water, herbal teas, and broths, to stay hydrated. This helps keep the respiratory tract moist and can soothe throat irritation.

2. **Avoid Irritants**:
   - Avoid exposure to smoke, pollutants, and other environmental irritants that can worsen cough symptoms.
   - Use a humidifier to add moisture to the air, especially in dry indoor environments, which can help ease coughing and soothe irritated airways.

3. **Rest and Sleep**:
   - Get adequate rest and prioritize sleep to support the body's immune system and promote healing.

4. **Nutritious Diet**:
   - Eat a balanced diet rich in fruits, vegetables, lean proteins, and whole grains to support overall health and immune function.
   - Include foods with anti-inflammatory properties, such as ginger, garlic, turmeric, and omega-3 fatty acids, which may help reduce inflammation in the respiratory tract.

5. **Avoid Trigger Foods**:
   - Limit or avoid foods that may exacerbate cough symptoms, such as spicy foods, acidic foods and beverages, dairy products, and processed or sugary foods.

6. **Gentle Exercise**:
   - Engage in gentle exercise, such as walking, yoga, or tai chi, to promote circulation and respiratory health.
   - Avoid strenuous exercise or activities that may exacerbate coughing or respiratory symptoms.

7. **Stress Management**:
   - Practice stress-reducing techniques, such as deep breathing exercises, meditation, or mindfulness, to help manage stress levels.

- Chronic stress can weaken the immune system and exacerbate cough symptoms, so finding healthy ways to cope with stress is important.

8. **Good Oral Hygiene**:
   - Maintain good oral hygiene by brushing and flossing regularly and using an alcohol-free mouthwash.
   - Oral health can impact respiratory health, so taking care of your teeth and gums may help reduce the risk of oral infections that could contribute to coughing.

9. **Avoid Alcohol and Caffeine**:
   - Limit or avoid alcohol and caffeine, as they can contribute to dehydration and may irritate the throat, worsening cough symptoms.

10. **Seek Medical Attention**:
    - If cough symptoms persist for more than a few weeks, are severe, or are accompanied by other concerning symptoms such as fever, difficulty breathing, or chest pain, seek medical attention promptly for proper diagnosis and treatment.

By incorporating these lifestyle and dietary considerations into your daily routine, you can help manage dry cough symptoms and support respiratory health. However, if cough symptoms persist or worsen despite these measures, it's important to consult with a healthcare professional for further evaluation and management.

Avoiding Irritants

Avoiding irritants is crucial for managing dry cough and maintaining respiratory health. Here are some key tips to minimize exposure to irritants:

1. **Quit Smoking**:
   - If you smoke, quitting is one of the most important steps you can take to protect your respiratory system. Smoking irritates the airways, leading to coughing and other respiratory symptoms.

2. **Avoid Secondhand Smoke**:
   - Limit exposure to secondhand smoke, which contains many of the same harmful chemicals as cigarette smoke and can irritate the respiratory tract.

3. **Reduce Indoor Air Pollution**:
   - Keep indoor air clean by using air purifiers or filters to remove pollutants, dust, and allergens.

- Ventilate your home regularly by opening windows and doors to allow fresh air to circulate.

4. **Minimize Exposure to Environmental Pollutants**:
   - Avoid spending time in areas with high levels of air pollution, such as near busy roads or industrial sites.
   - Check air quality reports and avoid outdoor activities on days when air pollution levels are high.

5. **Use Protective Equipment**:
   - If you work in environments with potential respiratory irritants, such as dust, chemicals, or fumes, use appropriate protective equipment such as masks or respirators.

6. **Reduce Allergen Exposure**:
   - Identify and minimize exposure to allergens that can trigger coughing, such as pollen, dust mites, pet dander, and mold.
   - Use allergen-proof covers on pillows and mattresses, and regularly clean bedding and carpets to reduce allergen buildup.

7. **Avoid Strong Odors and Perfumes**:
   - Strong odors and perfumes can irritate the respiratory tract and trigger coughing in sensitive

individuals. Avoid using or being around strong-smelling products whenever possible.

8. **Protect Against Indoor Irritants**:
   - Use non-toxic cleaning products and avoid using aerosol sprays or harsh chemicals that can release irritating fumes.
   - Keep indoor humidity levels between 30-50% to prevent mold growth and reduce respiratory irritation.

9. **Protect Against Outdoor Irritants**:
   - Wear a mask or scarf over your mouth and nose on cold or windy days to help warm and humidify the air before you breathe it in.
   - Avoid outdoor activities during times of high pollen or pollution levels, especially if you are prone to respiratory irritation.

10. **Stay Informed**:
    - Stay informed about potential irritants in your environment and take proactive steps to minimize exposure.
    - Monitor air quality reports, pollen counts, and other relevant information to make informed decisions about outdoor activities and exposure risks.

By avoiding respiratory irritants and minimizing exposure to potential triggers, you can help reduce the frequency and severity of dry cough episodes and support overall respiratory health. If you have specific concerns or questions about avoiding irritants, consult with a healthcare professional for personalized advice and guidance.

Dietary Modifications for Managing Dry Cough

Making dietary modifications can play a significant role in managing dry cough and supporting respiratory health. Here are some dietary tips to consider:

1. **Stay Hydrated**:
   - Drink plenty of fluids, such as water, herbal teas, and clear broths, to keep the respiratory tract moist and help thin mucus secretions, making them easier to expel through coughing.

2. **Consume Anti-inflammatory Foods**:
   - Include foods rich in anti-inflammatory nutrients, such as fruits, vegetables, whole grains, nuts, seeds, and fatty fish like salmon and mackerel.

- Incorporate foods with anti-inflammatory properties, such as ginger, turmeric, garlic, onions, and leafy greens, into your meals regularly.

3. **Include Vitamin C-Rich Foods**:
   - Vitamin C is known for its immune-boosting and antioxidant properties, which can help support respiratory health and reduce the severity of cough symptoms.
   - Include foods high in vitamin C, such as citrus fruits (oranges, lemons, grapefruits), kiwi, strawberries, bell peppers, and broccoli, in your diet.

4. **Increase Fluid Intake**:
   - Consume warm liquids like herbal teas, warm water with lemon and honey, and clear broths, which can help soothe the throat and provide relief from coughing.

5. **Avoid Trigger Foods**:
   - Limit or avoid foods and beverages that may exacerbate cough symptoms or trigger acid reflux, such as spicy foods, acidic foods and beverages (citrus fruits, tomatoes, coffee, carbonated drinks), dairy products, and processed or sugary foods.

6. **Incorporate Honey and Lemon**:
   - Honey has natural antibacterial and soothing properties that can help relieve throat irritation and suppress coughing. Stir honey into warm water or herbal teas for added relief.
   - Lemon is rich in vitamin C and can help thin mucus secretions, making them easier to expel. Squeeze fresh lemon juice into warm water or herbal teas for additional benefits.

7. **Choose Warm and Soothing Foods**:
   - Opt for warm, soothing foods such as soups, stews, oatmeal, and cooked grains, which can help provide comfort and relief from coughing.
   - Avoid foods and beverages that are too hot or too cold, as extreme temperatures can irritate the throat and trigger coughing.

8. **Moderate Alcohol and Caffeine Intake**:
   - Limit alcohol and caffeine consumption, as they can contribute to dehydration and may irritate the throat, worsening cough symptoms.

9. **Maintain a Balanced Diet**:
   - Eat a balanced diet that includes a variety of nutrient-dense foods to support overall health and immune function.

- Include lean proteins, healthy fats, and complex carbohydrates to provide essential nutrients and energy for optimal well-being.

10. **Listen to Your Body**:
   - Pay attention to how your body responds to different foods and beverages, and make adjustments accordingly.
   - If certain foods or drinks worsen cough symptoms or cause discomfort, consider eliminating or reducing them from your diet.

By making dietary modifications and choosing foods that support respiratory health, you can help manage dry cough symptoms and promote overall well-being. However, if cough symptoms persist or worsen despite dietary changes, it's essential to consult with a healthcare professional for further evaluation and management.

Proper Sleep Hygiene for Managing Dry Cough

Good sleep hygiene practices can contribute to better overall health and may help manage dry cough symptoms. Here are some tips for promoting restful sleep and reducing coughing at night:

1. **Establish a Consistent Sleep Schedule**:
   - Go to bed and wake up at the same time every day, even on weekends, to regulate your body's internal clock and promote better sleep quality.

2. **Create a Relaxing Bedtime Routine**:
   - Develop a calming pre-sleep routine to signal to your body that it's time to wind down. This could include activities such as reading, taking a warm bath, practicing relaxation techniques like deep breathing or meditation, or listening to soothing music.

3. **Create a Comfortable Sleep Environment**:
   - Make sure your bedroom is conducive to sleep by keeping it cool, dark, and quiet. Use blackout curtains, earplugs, or white noise machines if necessary to block out external disruptions.
   - Invest in a comfortable mattress and pillows that provide adequate support for your body.

4. **Avoid Stimulants Before Bed**:
   - Avoid consuming caffeine and nicotine in the hours leading up to bedtime, as they can interfere with your ability to fall asleep and stay asleep.
   - Limit alcohol intake, as it can disrupt sleep patterns and may worsen cough symptoms.

5. **Limit Screen Time Before Bed**:
   - Reduce exposure to electronic devices such as smartphones, tablets, computers, and televisions in the hour before bedtime. The blue light emitted by these devices can interfere with the production of melatonin, the hormone that regulates sleep.
   - Consider using blue light filters or "night mode" settings on electronic devices to reduce exposure to blue light in the evening.

6. **Address Allergens and Irritants**:
   - Keep your bedroom clean and free of dust, pet dander, and other allergens that can trigger coughing and disrupt sleep.
   - Use hypoallergenic bedding and pillow covers to minimize exposure to allergens.

7. **Elevate Your Head**:
   - If coughing worsens when lying flat, try elevating the head of your bed or using extra pillows to prop yourself up. This can help reduce postnasal drip and throat irritation.

8. **Stay Hydrated**:
   - Drink plenty of fluids throughout the day to stay hydrated, but try to limit intake in the hours leading up to bedtime to reduce the likelihood of needing to urinate during the night.

9. **Use Cough Remedies Before Bed**:
   - Take any prescribed or over-the-counter cough medications or remedies before bedtime as directed by your healthcare provider.
   - Use throat lozenges, cough syrups, or other cough suppressants to help reduce coughing and throat irritation during the night.

10. **Consult a Healthcare Professional**:
    - If coughing at night persists despite implementing sleep hygiene practices and using cough remedies, consult with a healthcare professional for further evaluation and treatment options.

By incorporating these sleep hygiene practices into your nightly routine, you can create a conducive environment for restful sleep and help minimize coughing episodes during the night. If coughing continues to disrupt your sleep or worsens over time, be sure to seek guidance from a healthcare professional for appropriate management and treatment.

Chapter 7

Professional Medical Treatment Options for Dry Cough

If home remedies and lifestyle modifications are not providing sufficient relief from dry cough, or if the cough is persistent or accompanied by other concerning symptoms, it may be necessary to seek medical treatment. Here are some professional medical treatment options for managing dry cough:

1. **Medical Evaluation**:
   - Consult with a healthcare professional, such as a primary care physician or pulmonologist, for a comprehensive evaluation of your cough symptoms.
   - Your healthcare provider will review your medical history, perform a physical examination, and may order diagnostic tests, such as chest X-rays, lung function tests, or blood tests, to determine the underlying cause of your cough.

2. **Prescription Medications**:
   - Depending on the underlying cause of the cough, your healthcare provider may prescribe medications to help alleviate symptoms and treat the underlying condition.

- For example, antibiotics may be prescribed for bacterial infections, corticosteroids may be used to reduce inflammation in the airways, and antihistamines or nasal corticosteroid sprays may be recommended for allergies or postnasal drip.

3. **Cough Suppressants**:
   - Prescription cough suppressants, such as codeine or dextromethorphan, may be prescribed to help reduce the frequency and intensity of coughing episodes, especially if the cough is interfering with sleep or daily activities.
   - These medications should be used with caution and under the guidance of a healthcare professional, as they can have side effects and may not be suitable for everyone.

4. **Bronchodilators**:
   - Bronchodilators, such as albuterol or ipratropium, may be prescribed to help open up the airways and improve breathing in individuals with asthma or chronic obstructive pulmonary disease (COPD) who are experiencing coughing and wheezing.

5. **Treatment of Underlying Conditions**:
   - If the dry cough is caused by an underlying medical condition, such as asthma, allergies,

gastroesophageal reflux disease (GERD), or chronic bronchitis, treatment will focus on managing and addressing the underlying condition.
  - This may involve lifestyle modifications, medication adjustments, or other interventions tailored to the specific condition contributing to the cough.

6. **Referral to Specialists**:
  - In some cases, your primary care physician may refer you to a specialist, such as a pulmonologist, allergist, gastroenterologist, or otolaryngologist, for further evaluation and management of your cough.
  - Specialists can provide expertise in diagnosing and treating respiratory, allergic, gastrointestinal, or throat-related conditions that may be contributing to the cough.

7. **Respiratory Therapy**:
  - Respiratory therapists can provide specialized treatments and techniques to help manage cough symptoms and improve respiratory function.
  - This may include pulmonary rehabilitation programs, breathing exercises, chest physiotherapy, or the use of airway clearance devices to help clear mucus from the lungs.

8. **Supportive Care**:
   - In addition to medical treatments, supportive care measures may be recommended to help alleviate symptoms and promote comfort.
   - This may include staying hydrated, using humidifiers or steam inhalation to moisturize the airways, and avoiding exposure to respiratory irritants or triggers.

It's important to work closely with your healthcare provider to develop an individualized treatment plan tailored to your specific needs and underlying condition. Be sure to follow your healthcare provider's recommendations and attend follow-up appointments as directed to monitor your progress and make any necessary adjustments to your treatment plan. If you experience any concerning or worsening symptoms, contact your healthcare provider promptly for further evaluation and management.

Prescription medications may be recommended by a healthcare professional to treat underlying conditions contributing to dry cough or to alleviate cough symptoms. Here are some common types of prescription medications used for managing dry cough:

1. **Antibiotics**:
   - If the dry cough is caused by a bacterial infection, such as pneumonia or bronchitis, antibiotics may be prescribed to target the underlying infection and reduce coughing.

2. **Corticosteroids**:
   - Corticosteroids, such as prednisone or fluticasone, may be prescribed to reduce inflammation in the airways and lungs, particularly in conditions like asthma or chronic obstructive pulmonary disease (COPD) that are associated with airway inflammation and coughing.

3. **Antihistamines**:
   - Antihistamines, such as cetirizine or loratadine, may be prescribed to treat allergies that contribute to cough symptoms by reducing allergic reactions and inflammation in the respiratory tract.

4. **Nasal Corticosteroid Sprays**:
   - Nasal corticosteroid sprays, such as fluticasone or mometasone, may be prescribed to reduce nasal congestion and postnasal drip, which can trigger coughing in individuals with allergic rhinitis or sinusitis.

5. **Bronchodilators**:
   - Bronchodilators, such as albuterol or tiotropium, may be prescribed to open up the airways and improve breathing in individuals with asthma, COPD, or other respiratory conditions associated with coughing and airway constriction.

6. **Proton Pump Inhibitors (PPIs)**:
   - Proton pump inhibitors, such as omeprazole or pantoprazole, may be prescribed to treat gastroesophageal reflux disease (GERD) and reduce stomach acid production, which can help alleviate coughing caused by acid reflux.

7. **ACE Inhibitors**:
   - ACE inhibitors, such as lisinopril or enalapril, are commonly used to treat high blood pressure and heart failure but can sometimes cause a persistent dry cough as a side effect. In such cases, switching to an alternative medication may be necessary.

8. **Opioid Cough Suppressants**:
   - Opioid-based cough suppressants, such as codeine or hydrocodone, may be prescribed for severe or persistent coughing that is not adequately controlled with other medications. These medications act on the brain to reduce the urge to cough.

9. **Immunosuppressants**:
   - In certain autoimmune conditions or chronic lung diseases, immunosuppressant medications such as azathioprine or methotrexate may be prescribed to reduce inflammation and suppress the immune response, thereby helping to alleviate cough symptoms.

10. **Mucolytics**:
    - Mucolytic medications, such as acetylcysteine or guaifenesin, may be prescribed to help thin and loosen mucus in the airways, making it easier to expel through coughing, particularly in individuals with chronic bronchitis or cystic fibrosis.

It's important to follow your healthcare provider's instructions carefully when taking prescription medications and to report any side effects or concerns promptly. Be sure to inform your healthcare provider about all medications, supplements, and over-the-counter drugs you are currently taking to avoid potential interactions or complications. Always use prescription medications as directed and attend follow-up appointments as recommended to monitor your progress and adjust your treatment plan as needed.

Immunotherapy for Managing Dry Cough

Immunotherapy, also known as allergy shots, is a treatment option primarily used for individuals with allergic conditions that contribute to chronic cough, such as allergic rhinitis (hay fever) or asthma. Here's how immunotherapy works and its potential benefits for managing dry cough:

1. **Targeting Allergen Sensitivity**:
   - Immunotherapy works by gradually desensitizing the immune system to specific allergens that trigger allergic reactions.
   - Allergy shots contain small amounts of allergens to which the individual is allergic. These allergens are administered in increasing doses over time to help the immune system build up tolerance.

2. **Reducing Allergic Responses**:
   - By exposing the immune system to gradually increasing amounts of allergens, immunotherapy helps reduce the body's exaggerated immune response to these allergens.
   - This can lead to a decrease in allergic symptoms, including nasal congestion, sneezing, wheezing, and coughing.

3. **Improving Respiratory Symptoms**:
   - For individuals with allergic asthma or allergic rhinitis, immunotherapy can help reduce airway inflammation and improve respiratory symptoms, including coughing.
   - By targeting the underlying allergic triggers, immunotherapy may lead to a reduction in cough frequency and severity over time.

4. **Long-Term Benefits**:
   - Immunotherapy is a long-term treatment approach that typically requires regular injections over several years to achieve maximum effectiveness.
   - Studies have shown that immunotherapy can provide long-lasting relief from allergic symptoms, even after treatment is discontinued.

5. **Customized Treatment Plans**:
   - Immunotherapy treatment plans are customized based on the individual's specific allergens and medical history.
   - Treatment typically begins with a build-up phase, during which injections are administered at increasing doses over several months, followed by a maintenance phase, during which injections are given at regular intervals to maintain tolerance.

6. **Supervised Treatment**:
   - Immunotherapy injections are administered under the supervision of a healthcare provider, usually in a clinical setting.
   - Patients are monitored closely for any adverse reactions, and adjustments to the treatment plan may be made as needed.

7. **Effectiveness for Allergic Conditions**:
   - Immunotherapy is most effective for individuals with allergic conditions caused by environmental allergens, such as pollen, dust mites, pet dander, or mold.
   - It may be less effective for non-allergic causes of cough, such as respiratory infections or irritant exposure.

8. **Consultation with an Allergist**:
   - If you suspect that allergies may be contributing to your chronic cough, consult with an allergist or immunologist for a comprehensive evaluation and discussion of treatment options.
   - Your healthcare provider can determine if immunotherapy is appropriate for your specific condition and develop a personalized treatment plan tailored to your needs.

Immunotherapy can be an effective treatment option for individuals with allergic conditions that contribute to chronic cough. By targeting the underlying allergic triggers, immunotherapy may help reduce cough frequency and severity over time, leading to improved respiratory health and overall quality of life.

Referral to a Specialist for Managing Dry Cough

When managing dry cough, a referral to a specialist may be necessary for further evaluation, diagnosis, and specialized treatment options. Here's how a referral to a specialist can benefit individuals with persistent or complex cough symptoms:

1. **Pulmonologist (Respiratory Specialist)**:
   - A pulmonologist is a physician who specializes in the diagnosis and treatment of respiratory conditions and diseases, including cough disorders.
   - A referral to a pulmonologist may be appropriate for individuals with chronic or unexplained cough that has not responded to initial treatments or is associated with respiratory conditions such as asthma, chronic obstructive pulmonary disease (COPD), interstitial lung disease, or bronchiectasis.

2. **Allergist/Immunologist**:
   - An allergist or immunologist specializes in the diagnosis and treatment of allergic conditions and immune system disorders.
   - A referral to an allergist or immunologist may be recommended for individuals with cough symptoms that are suspected to be related to allergies, such as allergic rhinitis (hay fever), allergic asthma, or hypersensitivity reactions to environmental triggers.

3. **Gastroenterologist**:
   - A gastroenterologist is a physician who specializes in the diagnosis and treatment of digestive system disorders, including gastroesophageal reflux disease (GERD) and gastrointestinal reflux-related cough.
   - A referral to a gastroenterologist may be warranted for individuals with chronic cough that is suspected to be caused or exacerbated by GERD or other esophageal disorders.

4. **Otolaryngologist (Ear, Nose, and Throat Specialist)**:
   - An otolaryngologist specializes in the diagnosis and treatment of disorders of the ear, nose, throat, and related structures.

- A referral to an otolaryngologist may be necessary for individuals with chronic cough that is suspected to be related to throat or laryngeal conditions, such as laryngopharyngeal reflux (LPR), vocal cord dysfunction, or chronic throat irritation.

5. **Infectious Disease Specialist**:
  - An infectious disease specialist is a physician who specializes in the diagnosis and treatment of infectious diseases caused by bacteria, viruses, fungi, or parasites.
  - A referral to an infectious disease specialist may be appropriate for individuals with cough symptoms that are suspected to be caused by underlying infections, such as pneumonia, tuberculosis, or fungal lung infections.

6. **Rheumatologist**:
  - A rheumatologist is a physician who specializes in the diagnosis and treatment of autoimmune and inflammatory disorders, including connective tissue diseases that may affect the lungs and cause cough symptoms.
  - A referral to a rheumatologist may be considered for individuals with cough symptoms that are suspected to be related to underlying autoimmune conditions, such as rheumatoid arthritis, systemic lupus erythematosus, or sarcoidosis.

7. **Neurologist**:
   - In rare cases, cough symptoms may be caused by neurological conditions affecting the nerves that control cough reflexes.
   - A referral to a neurologist may be necessary for individuals with chronic cough that is suspected to be related to neurological disorders, such as stroke, Parkinson's disease, or multiple sclerosis.

8. **Multidisciplinary Approach**:
   - In some cases, a multidisciplinary approach involving collaboration between different specialists may be beneficial for comprehensive evaluation and management of complex cough disorders.
   - Your primary care physician can coordinate referrals and facilitate communication between specialists to ensure coordinated care and optimize treatment outcomes.

By referring individuals with persistent or complex cough symptoms to appropriate specialists, healthcare providers can ensure that patients receive comprehensive evaluation, accurate diagnosis, and tailored treatment plans to address the underlying causes of their cough and improve their overall respiratory health and quality of life.

Chapter 8

Prevention Strategies for Managing Dry Cough

Preventing dry cough involves minimizing exposure to irritants, addressing underlying health conditions, and adopting healthy lifestyle habits. Here are some prevention strategies to consider:

1. **Avoid Respiratory Irritants**:
   - Minimize exposure to tobacco smoke, air pollution, dust, and other environmental irritants that can trigger coughing.
   - Use air purifiers or filters in your home to remove allergens and pollutants from the air.

2. **Practice Good Hygiene**:
   - Wash your hands frequently with soap and water to reduce the spread of respiratory infections.
   - Cover your mouth and nose with a tissue or your elbow when coughing or sneezing to prevent the spread of germs.

3. **Manage Underlying Health Conditions**:
   - Follow your healthcare provider's recommendations for managing underlying health

conditions that can contribute to coughing, such as asthma, allergies, GERD, or chronic bronchitis.
   - Take prescribed medications as directed and attend regular follow-up appointments to monitor your condition and adjust treatment as needed.

4. **Stay Hydrated**:
   - Drink plenty of fluids throughout the day to keep your respiratory tract moist and help thin mucus secretions, making them easier to expel through coughing.

5. **Practice Good Sleep Hygiene**:
   - Maintain a regular sleep schedule, create a relaxing bedtime routine, and ensure your sleep environment is comfortable and conducive to restful sleep.
   - Elevate your head while sleeping if coughing worsens at night, using extra pillows or an adjustable bed.

6. **Manage Stress**:
   - Practice stress-reducing techniques such as deep breathing, meditation, yoga, or progressive muscle relaxation to help reduce stress levels, which can exacerbate coughing.

7. **Stay Active and Exercise Regularly**:
   - Engage in regular physical activity to support respiratory health and immune function.
   - Choose activities that you enjoy and can incorporate into your daily routine, such as walking, cycling, swimming, or yoga.

8. **Maintain a Healthy Diet**:
   - Eat a balanced diet rich in fruits, vegetables, whole grains, lean proteins, and healthy fats to support overall health and immune function.
   - Limit intake of processed foods, sugary snacks, and beverages high in caffeine or alcohol, which can exacerbate coughing and inflammation.

9. **Quit Smoking**:
   - If you smoke, quit smoking to reduce your risk of developing respiratory conditions and coughing-related complications.
   - Seek support from healthcare professionals, smoking cessation programs, or support groups to help you quit successfully.

10. **Stay Informed and Seek Medical Advice**:
    - Stay informed about respiratory health, common causes of coughing, and preventive measures you can take to protect yourself.

- Consult with a healthcare professional if you experience persistent or worsening cough symptoms, especially if accompanied by other concerning symptoms such as fever, chest pain, or difficulty breathing.

By incorporating these prevention strategies into your daily routine and lifestyle, you can help minimize your risk of developing dry cough and maintain optimal respiratory health. If you have specific concerns or underlying health conditions, consult with a healthcare professional for personalized advice and guidance on preventive measures.

Hand Hygiene for Preventing Dry Cough

Maintaining good hand hygiene is essential for preventing the spread of respiratory infections that can lead to dry cough. Here are some key practices to follow:

1. **Handwashing Technique**:
   - Wash your hands frequently with soap and water for at least 20 seconds, especially after coughing, sneezing, blowing your nose, or touching surfaces in public places.

- Rub your hands together vigorously, covering all surfaces, including the backs of your hands, between your fingers, and under your nails.

- Rinse your hands thoroughly under running water and dry them with a clean towel or air dryer.

2. **Use of Hand Sanitizer**:

- When soap and water are not readily available, use an alcohol-based hand sanitizer containing at least 60% alcohol.

- Apply a sufficient amount of sanitizer to the palm of one hand and rub your hands together, covering all surfaces until dry.

- Hand sanitizers are effective at killing many types of germs, but they may not be as effective as soap and water against certain viruses, such as norovirus.

3. **Avoid Touching Your Face**:

- Avoid touching your eyes, nose, and mouth with unwashed hands, as these are common entry points for germs to enter your body and cause respiratory infections.

- Encourage children to avoid touching their face and mouth to reduce their risk of contracting respiratory illnesses.

4. **Hand Hygiene in Public Places**:
   - Practice hand hygiene when using public transportation, shopping, dining out, or engaging in other activities outside the home.
   - Use hand sanitizing wipes or gel before and after touching surfaces such as doorknobs, handrails, elevator buttons, shopping carts, and touchscreen kiosks.

5. **Handwashing Before Eating or Handling Food**:
   - Wash your hands thoroughly with soap and water before preparing or eating food, as well as after handling raw meat, poultry, or eggs.
   - Proper hand hygiene can help prevent the transmission of foodborne pathogens that can cause gastrointestinal infections and other illnesses.

6. **Hand Hygiene at Work and School**:
   - Encourage hand hygiene practices in the workplace and educational settings by providing access to handwashing facilities, hand sanitizer, and educational materials on proper handwashing techniques.
   - Encourage employees, students, and visitors to stay home if they are sick to prevent the spread of illness to others.

7. **Lead by Example**:
   - Set a positive example by practicing good hand hygiene habits yourself and reinforcing the importance of handwashing with your family, friends, and colleagues.
   - Make handwashing a routine part of your daily activities and encourage others to do the same.

By practicing regular hand hygiene, you can help reduce your risk of contracting respiratory infections and prevent the spread of germs to others, ultimately contributing to a healthier environment for everyone.

Vaccinations for Preventing Dry Cough and Respiratory Infections

Vaccinations play a crucial role in preventing dry cough and reducing the risk of respiratory infections caused by viruses and bacteria. Here are some key vaccinations recommended for preventing respiratory illnesses:

1. **Influenza (Flu) Vaccine**:
   - The seasonal influenza vaccine helps protect against the flu virus, which can cause symptoms such as cough, fever, sore throat, and body aches.

- Annual flu vaccination is recommended for everyone aged six months and older, especially individuals at higher risk of complications, including young children, older adults, pregnant women, and individuals with underlying health conditions.

2. **Pneumococcal Vaccine**:
   - Pneumococcal vaccines protect against infections caused by the bacterium Streptococcus pneumoniae, which can lead to pneumonia, bronchitis, and other respiratory illnesses.
   - Different pneumococcal vaccines are recommended for different age groups and risk factors. Adults aged 65 years and older and individuals with certain medical conditions may require pneumococcal vaccination.

3. **COVID-19 Vaccine**:
   - COVID-19 vaccines are designed to protect against the severe acute respiratory syndrome coronavirus 2 (SARS-CoV-2), which causes COVID-19.
   - Vaccination against COVID-19 is recommended for everyone eligible for vaccination, including adolescents and adults, to reduce the risk of infection, severe illness, and transmission of the virus.

4. **Tdap and Td Vaccines**:
   - The Tdap vaccine protects against tetanus, diphtheria, and pertussis (whooping cough), while the Td vaccine protects against tetanus and diphtheria.
   - Tdap vaccination is recommended for adolescents and adults to protect against pertussis and prevent the spread of whooping cough to vulnerable populations, such as infants who are too young to be fully vaccinated.

5. **Measles, Mumps, and Rubella (MMR) Vaccine**:
   - The MMR vaccine protects against measles, mumps, and rubella viruses, which can cause respiratory symptoms along with other complications.
   - Vaccination against measles, mumps, and rubella is recommended for children and adults who have not previously been vaccinated or are not immune to these diseases.

6. **Varicella (Chickenpox) Vaccine**:
   - The varicella vaccine protects against the varicella-zoster virus, which causes chickenpox, a contagious viral infection characterized by fever, rash, and respiratory symptoms.

- Vaccination against chickenpox is recommended for children and adults who have not had the disease or been vaccinated against it.

7. **Other Vaccines**:
   - Depending on individual risk factors, travel plans, and medical history, other vaccines may be recommended to prevent respiratory infections and related complications. These may include vaccines against hepatitis A and B, meningococcal disease, and Haemophilus influenzae type b (Hib).

It's essential to stay up-to-date with recommended vaccinations according to national guidelines and consult with healthcare providers to determine which vaccines are appropriate based on age, medical history, occupation, travel plans, and other factors. Vaccinations not only protect individuals from respiratory infections but also help prevent the spread of infectious diseases within communities, contributing to public health and well-being.

Avoiding Exposure to Allergens and Irritants to Prevent Dry Cough

Minimizing exposure to allergens and irritants is crucial for preventing dry cough, especially in individuals prone to respiratory allergies or sensitivities. Here are some strategies to avoid exposure to common allergens and irritants:

1. **Identify Allergens**:
    - Work with an allergist to identify specific allergens that trigger your cough symptoms. Common allergens include pollen, dust mites, pet dander, mold spores, and certain foods.

2. **Monitor Pollen Counts**:
    - Stay informed about pollen counts in your area, especially during peak allergy seasons. Limit outdoor activities on high pollen days, particularly in the morning when pollen levels are typically highest.

3. **Keep Indoor Air Clean**:
    - Use high-efficiency particulate air (HEPA) filters in your home's heating and cooling systems to trap airborne allergens like pollen, dust, and pet dander.
    - Regularly vacuum carpets, rugs, and upholstered furniture using a vacuum cleaner equipped with a

HEPA filter to remove allergens from indoor surfaces.

4. **Control Dust Mites**:
   - Encase mattresses, pillows, and box springs in allergen-proof covers to prevent dust mites from accumulating in bedding.
   - Wash bedding, including sheets, pillowcases, and blankets, in hot water (130°F or higher) weekly to kill dust mites and remove allergens.

5. **Reduce Pet Allergens**:
   - Limit exposure to pet allergens by keeping pets out of bedrooms and off upholstered furniture.
   - Bathe pets regularly and groom them outdoors to reduce dander and allergens in the home.

6. **Prevent Mold Growth**:
   - Keep indoor humidity levels between 30% and 50% to inhibit mold growth. Use a dehumidifier if necessary, especially in damp areas like basements and bathrooms.
   - Fix water leaks promptly and ensure proper ventilation in bathrooms, kitchens, and laundry areas to prevent moisture buildup.

7. **Avoid Tobacco Smoke**:
   - Avoid exposure to tobacco smoke, whether firsthand or secondhand, as it can exacerbate cough symptoms and respiratory irritation.
   - If you smoke, quit smoking, and avoid environments where smoking is permitted to protect your respiratory health.

8. **Minimize Exposure to Strong Odors and Chemicals**:
   - Avoid exposure to strong odors, perfumes, cleaning products, and household chemicals that can irritate the respiratory tract and trigger coughing.
   - Use natural or fragrance-free cleaning products and air fresheners to minimize exposure to harsh chemicals and volatile organic compounds (VOCs).

9. **Wear Protective Gear**:
   - When engaging in outdoor activities that may expose you to allergens or irritants, such as gardening or yard work, wear a mask or respirator to filter out airborne particles and protect your airways.

10. **Monitor Indoor Air Quality**:
    - Test your home for indoor air pollutants, such as radon, carbon monoxide, and volatile organic

compounds (VOCs), and take steps to mitigate any sources of indoor air pollution.

By taking proactive measures to avoid exposure to allergens and irritants, you can help prevent dry cough and minimize respiratory symptoms associated with allergic reactions and environmental sensitivities. If symptoms persist despite avoidance measures or worsen over time, consult with a healthcare professional for further evaluation and management.

Chapter 9

When to Seek Medical Attention

Knowing when to seek medical attention for a dry cough is important to ensure timely diagnosis and appropriate treatment. Here are some signs and symptoms that indicate it may be time to consult a healthcare professional:

1. **Persistent Cough**: If your cough persists for more than three weeks and does not improve with home remedies or over-the-counter treatments, it's essential to seek medical advice.

2. **Severe Coughing Spells**: If you experience severe or uncontrollable coughing spells that interfere with your ability to breathe, speak, or sleep, seek immediate medical attention, as this could indicate a more serious underlying condition.

3. **Coughing Up Blood**: If you cough up blood or notice blood in your sputum (mucus), it's important to see a healthcare provider promptly, as this could be a sign of a serious medical problem, such as pneumonia, bronchitis, tuberculosis, or lung cancer.

4. **Difficulty Breathing**: If you experience difficulty breathing, shortness of breath, wheezing, or chest tightness along with your cough, seek medical attention immediately, as these symptoms could indicate a potentially life-threatening condition, such as asthma exacerbation, pulmonary embolism, or heart failure.

5. **Fever**: If you develop a fever along with your cough, especially if it is high or persistent, it may indicate an underlying infection that requires medical evaluation and treatment.

6. **Other Symptoms**: If your cough is accompanied by other concerning symptoms, such as chest pain, fatigue, weight loss, night sweats, or swollen lymph nodes, it's important to see a healthcare provider for a thorough evaluation to determine the underlying cause.

7. **Underlying Health Conditions**: If you have underlying health conditions, such as asthma, chronic obstructive pulmonary disease (COPD), gastroesophageal reflux disease (GERD), or immune system disorders, and your cough worsens or is not responding to treatment, consult with your healthcare provider for appropriate management.

8. **Recent Travel or Exposure**: If you have recently traveled to areas with a high incidence of respiratory infections or have been in close contact with individuals who have respiratory symptoms, and you develop a cough, it's advisable to seek medical advice to rule out infectious causes.

9. **Persistent Symptoms**: If you experience persistent symptoms such as fatigue, weakness, loss of appetite, or malaise along with your cough, consult with a healthcare provider for further evaluation, as these symptoms may indicate an underlying systemic illness.

10. **Concern for COVID-19**: If you develop symptoms consistent with COVID-19, such as cough, fever, shortness of breath, loss of taste or smell, or muscle aches, get tested for COVID-19 and follow public health guidelines for isolation and medical care.

If you are unsure whether your symptoms warrant medical attention, it's always best to err on the side of caution and consult with a healthcare professional for guidance. Prompt evaluation and treatment can help prevent complications and ensure the best possible outcome for your respiratory health.

If you experience persistent or severe symptoms associated with a dry cough, it's important to seek medical attention promptly. Here's why:

1. **Underlying Conditions**: Persistent or severe symptoms may indicate an underlying medical condition that requires evaluation and treatment by a healthcare professional. Conditions such as asthma, chronic bronchitis, pneumonia, or even lung cancer can present with persistent or severe coughing.

2. **Complications**: Ignoring persistent or severe symptoms can lead to complications. For example, untreated respiratory infections can progress to more serious conditions such as pneumonia, bronchitis, or respiratory failure. Early intervention can prevent complications and improve outcomes.

3. **Quality of Life**: Persistent or severe coughing can significantly impact your quality of life by disrupting sleep, impairing daily activities, and causing discomfort or distress. Seeking medical attention can help alleviate symptoms and improve your overall well-being.

4. **Risk of Transmission**: In cases where the cough is due to an infectious cause, such as a cold,

flu, or COVID-19, prompt medical attention can help reduce the risk of spreading the infection to others. Taking appropriate precautions and receiving timely treatment can help limit transmission within your household and community.

5. **Diagnostic Evaluation**: A healthcare professional can conduct a thorough evaluation to determine the underlying cause of your symptoms. This may involve a physical examination, medical history review, diagnostic tests (such as chest X-rays or pulmonary function tests), and other assessments to identify the underlying condition contributing to your cough.

6. **Treatment Options**: Once the underlying cause of your cough is identified, appropriate treatment options can be recommended. This may include medications, lifestyle modifications, breathing exercises, or other interventions tailored to your specific needs and condition.

7. **Monitoring and Follow-Up**: Seeking medical attention allows for ongoing monitoring of your symptoms and response to treatment. Your healthcare provider can adjust your treatment plan

as needed and provide follow-up care to ensure your symptoms are effectively managed over time.

Remember that persistent or severe symptoms should not be ignored, as they may indicate an underlying health issue that requires attention. By seeking medical help promptly, you can receive the appropriate care and support needed to address your symptoms and improve your respiratory health.

Dry cough itself is not typically considered a serious medical condition, but it can be a symptom of an underlying health issue. While dry cough may not directly cause complications, the conditions that lead to persistent or severe coughing can result in various complications. Here are some potential complications associated with underlying causes of dry cough:

1. **Respiratory Infections**: If the dry cough is caused by a respiratory infection such as bronchitis, pneumonia, or influenza, complications can include:
   - Severe respiratory symptoms such as difficulty breathing or shortness of breath.

- Pneumonia, especially in vulnerable populations such as young children, older adults, or individuals with weakened immune systems.
- Acute respiratory distress syndrome (ARDS), a life-threatening condition characterized by severe lung inflammation and fluid buildup in the air sacs.

2. **Asthma**: Individuals with asthma may experience complications such as:
- Asthma exacerbations or attacks characterized by severe coughing, wheezing, chest tightness, and difficulty breathing.
- Respiratory failure, particularly during severe asthma attacks, which can be life-threatening without prompt medical intervention.

3. **Chronic Obstructive Pulmonary Disease (COPD)**: Complications associated with COPD and chronic bronchitis may include:
- Exacerbations of COPD, marked by worsening cough, increased sputum production, and shortness of breath.
- Respiratory infections, which can lead to further lung damage and exacerbate COPD symptoms.
- Pulmonary hypertension, a condition characterized by high blood pressure in the arteries of the lungs, which can strain the heart and impair lung function.

4. **Gastroesophageal Reflux Disease (GERD)**: Chronic cough due to GERD can result in complications such as:
   - Esophageal inflammation or irritation, which may lead to complications such as esophagitis, esophageal strictures, or Barrett's esophagus.
   - Respiratory complications such as aspiration pneumonia, in which stomach contents are inhaled into the lungs, leading to lung infection or inflammation.

5. **Lung Cancer**: A persistent dry cough can be a symptom of lung cancer, and complications may include:
   - Advanced-stage lung cancer with metastasis (spread) to other organs, leading to systemic complications and reduced survival rates.
   - Complications related to cancer treatment, such as chemotherapy, radiation therapy, or surgery, including side effects such as infection, fatigue, or respiratory issues.

6. **Psychosocial Impact**: Chronic cough can have a significant psychosocial impact, leading to complications such as:
   - Sleep disturbances, including insomnia or daytime sleepiness, which can impair cognitive function, mood, and overall quality of life.

- Social isolation or withdrawal due to embarrassment or discomfort associated with persistent coughing in public settings.

It's important to address underlying causes of dry cough promptly to prevent complications and improve respiratory health. If you experience persistent or severe coughing, consult with a healthcare professional for evaluation, diagnosis, and appropriate treatment. Early intervention can help mitigate complications and improve outcomes.

Dry cough can be a symptom of various underlying health conditions affecting the respiratory system, gastrointestinal tract, or immune system. Here are some common underlying health conditions associated with dry cough:

1. **Respiratory Infections**:
   - **Common Cold**: Viral infections such as the common cold can cause irritation of the upper respiratory tract, leading to a dry cough.
   - **Influenza (Flu)**: Influenza viruses can cause respiratory symptoms including cough, fever, sore throat, and body aches.
   - **Bronchitis**: Acute bronchitis, often caused by viral infections, is characterized by inflammation of

the bronchial tubes and can lead to a persistent dry cough.

   - **Pneumonia**: Bacterial or viral pneumonia can cause inflammation and fluid buildup in the lungs, resulting in coughing, fever, and difficulty breathing.

2. **Asthma**:
   - **Allergic Asthma**: In individuals with allergic asthma, exposure to allergens such as pollen, dust mites, or pet dander can trigger airway inflammation and bronchospasm, leading to coughing and wheezing.
   - **Non-Allergic Asthma**: Non-allergic asthma triggers may include respiratory infections, exercise, cold air, or irritants such as smoke or pollution.

3. **Chronic Obstructive Pulmonary Disease (COPD)**:
   - **Chronic Bronchitis**: COPD, particularly chronic bronchitis, is characterized by persistent inflammation of the bronchial tubes, excessive mucus production, and a chronic, productive cough.
   - **Emphysema**: Emphysema is characterized by damage to the air sacs in the lungs, leading to

airflow limitation and respiratory symptoms such as coughing and shortness of breath.

4. **Gastroesophageal Reflux Disease (GERD)**:
   - GERD occurs when stomach acid flows back into the esophagus, leading to irritation and inflammation of the esophageal lining. Chronic cough due to GERD is often worse after eating or when lying down and may be associated with heartburn or regurgitation.

5. **Postnasal Drip**:
   - Postnasal drip occurs when excess mucus from the nasal passages drips down the back of the throat, leading to irritation and coughing. It can be caused by allergies, sinus infections, or environmental irritants.

6. **Interstitial Lung Diseases**:
   - Conditions such as idiopathic pulmonary fibrosis (IPF), sarcoidosis, or connective tissue diseases can cause inflammation and scarring of lung tissue, leading to coughing and difficulty breathing.

7. **Medication Side Effects**:
   - Certain medications, such as angiotensin-converting enzyme (ACE) inhibitors

used to treat hypertension, can cause a persistent dry cough as a side effect.

8. **Lung Cancer**:
   - Lung cancer, particularly non-small cell lung cancer, can cause symptoms such as persistent cough, chest pain, shortness of breath, and coughing up blood.

9. **Allergic Rhinitis (Hay Fever)**:
   - Allergic rhinitis can cause nasal congestion, postnasal drip, and throat irritation, leading to coughing, particularly at night or upon waking.

10. **Immunodeficiency Disorders**:
    - Conditions that weaken the immune system, such as HIV/AIDS or immunodeficiency syndromes, can increase the risk of respiratory infections and chronic cough.

If you experience persistent or severe dry cough, it's important to consult with a healthcare professional for evaluation and appropriate management. Identifying and treating the underlying health condition is essential for relieving symptoms and improving respiratory health.

Conclusion

In conclusion, dry cough is a common symptom that can be caused by various underlying health conditions affecting the respiratory system, gastrointestinal tract, or immune system. While occasional dry cough is often benign and resolves on its own, persistent or severe coughing may indicate an underlying medical issue that requires evaluation and treatment.

Understanding the potential causes of dry cough, including respiratory infections, asthma, COPD, GERD, and others, is essential for effective management and prevention of complications. Prompt identification and treatment of underlying health conditions can help alleviate symptoms, improve respiratory health, and prevent complications.

In addition to medical interventions, lifestyle modifications such as avoiding allergens and irritants, practicing good hand hygiene, staying hydrated, and maintaining proper sleep hygiene can help reduce the frequency and severity of dry cough episodes.

If you experience persistent or severe dry cough, or if your cough is accompanied by other concerning symptoms such as difficulty breathing, coughing up blood, or fever, it's important to seek medical attention for a thorough evaluation and appropriate management.

By understanding the potential causes and risk factors associated with dry cough, individuals can take proactive steps to protect their respiratory health, improve quality of life, and reduce the risk of complications associated with underlying health conditions. With timely intervention and proper management, many cases of dry cough can be effectively treated, leading to symptom relief and improved overall well-being.

Here's a summary of the key points regarding dry cough and its management:

1. **Definition and Characteristics**:
   - Dry cough is a type of cough that does not produce phlegm or mucus and is often characterized by a tickling or irritation in the throat.

2. **Causes of Dry Cough**:
   - Common causes include respiratory infections, asthma, allergies, GERD, COPD, medications, and environmental irritants.

3. **Common Symptoms**:
   - Symptoms may include persistent coughing, throat irritation, hoarseness, chest discomfort, and difficulty breathing.

4. **Importance of Treatment**:
   - Treating dry cough is important to alleviate symptoms, prevent complications, and improve quality of life.

5. **Impact on Quality of Life**:
   - Dry cough can significantly impact daily activities, sleep quality, and overall well-being if left untreated.

6. **Complications of Untreated Dry Cough**:
   - Complications may include respiratory infections, exacerbation of underlying conditions, and psychosocial effects.

7. **Home Remedies**:
   - Hydration, herbal teas, honey and lemon, steam inhalation, gargling with salt water, throat lozenges,

humidifiers, breathing exercises, and dietary modifications can help relieve dry cough.

8. **Over-the-Counter Medications**:
   - Antitussives, expectorants, decongestants, analgesics, and NSAIDs may provide relief for certain types of dry cough.

9. **Natural Supplements and Herbs**:
   - Echinacea, ginger, marshmallow root, slippery elm, and licorice root are among the natural supplements and herbs that may help alleviate cough symptoms.

10. **Lifestyle and Dietary Considerations**:
    - Avoiding irritants, maintaining proper sleep hygiene, and adopting a healthy diet can contribute to managing dry cough.

11. **Professional Medical Treatment Options**:
    - Prescription medications, immunotherapy, referral to specialists, and vaccinations may be recommended for managing underlying conditions associated with dry cough.

12. **Hand Hygiene**:
   - Practicing good hand hygiene can help prevent the spread of respiratory infections and reduce the risk of cough transmission.

13. **When to Seek Medical Attention**:
   - Seek medical attention for persistent or severe coughing, coughing up blood, difficulty breathing, fever, or other concerning symptoms.

14. **Summary of Underlying Health Conditions**:
   - Respiratory infections, asthma, COPD, GERD, postnasal drip, interstitial lung diseases, medication side effects, lung cancer, allergic rhinitis, and immunodeficiency disorders are common underlying causes of dry cough.

15. **Conclusion**:
   - Understanding the causes and management strategies for dry cough is essential for effective treatment, symptom relief, and prevention of complications.

By addressing underlying causes, adopting appropriate management strategies, and seeking medical attention when necessary, individuals can effectively manage dry cough and improve their respiratory health and quality of life.

Seeking appropriate treatment for your dry cough is essential for your overall health and well-being. Here's some encouragement to take that important step:

1. **Relief from Discomfort**: By seeking treatment, you can alleviate the discomfort and irritation caused by your dry cough. Whether it's persistent tickling in your throat or frequent coughing fits disrupting your daily life, proper treatment can offer relief and improve your comfort.

2. **Prevention of Complications**: Addressing the underlying cause of your dry cough can help prevent potential complications. Untreated respiratory infections, asthma exacerbations, or other underlying conditions may lead to more severe health issues if left untreated. Seeking appropriate treatment early can help prevent these complications from arising.

3. **Improvement in Quality of Life**: Chronic coughing can take a toll on your quality of life, affecting your ability to sleep, work, socialize, and

enjoy daily activities. By seeking treatment, you can regain control over your symptoms and improve your overall quality of life.

4. **Customized Care**: Healthcare professionals can provide personalized care tailored to your specific needs and medical history. They can assess your symptoms, perform necessary tests or evaluations, and recommend a treatment plan that addresses the root cause of your dry cough, ensuring the most effective outcome.

5. **Empowerment through Knowledge**: Seeking medical attention allows you to gain a better understanding of your condition and the factors contributing to your dry cough. With knowledge comes empowerment—you'll be better equipped to manage your symptoms, make informed decisions about your health, and take proactive steps to prevent future episodes.

6. **Support and Guidance**: You don't have to face your dry cough alone. Healthcare professionals are there to offer support, guidance, and reassurance throughout your treatment journey. Whether you need advice on lifestyle modifications, assistance with medication management, or emotional support, they're here to help.

7. **Investment in Long-Term Health**: Taking the initiative to seek appropriate treatment for your dry cough is an investment in your long-term health. By addressing underlying health issues and managing your symptoms effectively, you can safeguard your respiratory health and enjoy a higher quality of life in the years to come.

Remember, your health and well-being are worth prioritizing. Don't hesitate to reach out to a healthcare professional for help with your dry cough. By seeking appropriate treatment, you're taking an important step toward a healthier, happier future.

www.ingramcontent.com/pod-product-compliance
Lightning Source LLC
Chambersburg PA
CBHW050304230526
45471CB00005B/2007